The Psychology of the Arab

The Psychology of the Arab

The Influences That Shape an Arab Life

Dr. Talib Kafaji

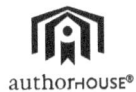

authorHOUSE®

AuthorHouse™
1663 Liberty Drive
Bloomington, IN 47403
www.authorhouse.com
Phone: 1-800-839-8640

First published by AuthorHouse   08/19/2011

ISBN: 978-1-4634-6821-7 (sc)
ISBN: 978-1-4634-6819-4 (hc)
ISBN: 978-1-4634-6820-0 (ebk)

Library of Congress Control Number: 2011914575

Printed in the United States of America

Any people depicted in stock imagery provided by Thinkstock are models, and such images are being used for illustrative purposes only.
Certain stock imagery © Thinkstock.

This book is printed on acid-free paper.

Because of the dynamic nature of the Internet, any web addresses or links contained in this book may have changed since publication and may no longer be valid. The views expressed in this work are solely those of the author and do not necessarily reflect the views of the publisher, and the publisher hereby disclaims any responsibility for them.

Contents

Introduction

A few years ago I was reading "The Arab Mind" by Raphael Pattie. I thought, I am the one who should write such a book, because the book deals specifically with the psychology of the Arab. I am a psychologist born in the Arab world but who lives, was educated and works in the United States. Perhaps I am in a better position to write about the Arab mind and psychology. I have been collecting a great deal of materials all these years to equip myself for this perilous adventure. I definitely am unable to give an impartial picture about the Arab psychology because I spent most of my adult life in my beloved adopted country of America.

Moreover, writing about the Arab psychology is a very difficult task, and I am sure I will open myself to all kinds of attacks and criticisms, because I am not going to be able to satisfy everyone. As the old wisdom goes, if two people look at the same thing, they will see it differently. There will be people, I am sure, who will be offended, and who want always to present a positive picture about Arab society. They do not want anyone to portray anything other than a rosy picture of the Arab world. As is said in the old expression, do not burst the bubbles that the Arab has put himself in for such a long time, just keep things bright and wonderful. Undoubtedly self-reflection in Arab culture is not encouraged; this is why they have stayed the way they are. However, I would say the "ostrich mentality" is definitely not helpful today.

However, I am venturing out and writing about the Arab psychology because I am a psychologist who worked for thirty years in the West, as well as in the Middle East. I am inviting the community of behavioral scientists to open a dialogue and have a critical mind to examine together the psychology of the Arab, and make this attempt beneficial to the Arab mind and psyche. Nevertheless, this is an attempt to shed some light on entire cultural practices, and see which ones can be valuable to the whole culture and should be reinforced, and which practices can be a hindrance and a barrier to moving forward toward a global development. This book is an investigation of the Arab culture, to see whether it is able to evolve and adapt to modern life, or if it is still holding onto archaic ways of thinking.

This book is not an attack on the Arab culture by any means. It is an attempt to bring to the attention of Arab individuals some insights into the causes of their behaviors. Once there is an insight then an individual can identify the weaknesses and strengths of their cultural practices, so he can reinforce the good and healthy, and weed out the dysfunctional and neurotic.

I am also attempting to bring to light the positive sides of these cultural practices, so that we may use them as antidotes to speed healing and recovery from a painful reality. Perhaps, sometimes I may fail to accentuate the positive practices of the culture. However, this is not out of malicious purpose, it is simply overlooked or inadvertent on my part, or it might be my unconscious biases. Whether we like it or not, these biases are beyond our control or conscious awareness.

I am writing this project out of my responsibility to the culture and for no other reason. It is a project I hope may stimulate some debate and raise more questions then answers. My aim is to plant the seed of self-examination, hoping that some readers may take it seriously and try to move the culture in the direction of evolution and liberation from self-made bondage.

I am also inviting the reader to put aside the subjectivity of your judgment, and try to see this look at psychological interpretations of Arabs through naked eyes. Once you have, then you will benefit from this book. I am sure some interpretations may sound too harsh or difficult to digest. Although, I would say there is nothing wrong in having an eagle eye to spot some of the pathology in Arab behaviors. Hence, I never claim to know it all; I am just an investigator in the science of human behavior.

We must also know that Arabs are like everybody else in that they are not totally good or totally bad by nature. They have both the higher self and the lower self as we can see in the coming chapters of the book, and the **caveat** here is, when I say "the Arab people", I mean specifically the majority of the people, not the total population. (For example, if we say the Japanese are industrious people, it does not mean there are no lazy people in Japan, but that the majority of them are industrious). The Holy book, the Quran, always talks about the majority of people being in darkness, or the majority of people are nonbelievers . . . and so on.

I know there are wonderful Arab people who have in their heart the sincere intention to contribute to the welfare of their community. Unfortunately, their voices are often not heard, and they are often run over by the opportunistic and hypocritical segments of society.

The Arab countries are rich with an abundance of natural resources, and more importantly healthy young populations. In spite of this, they lag behind many other countries around the world. What is needed in the Arab world is a look deep inside the dynamic of culture and the contributions that have shaped individuals' perspective positively or negatively. More importantly, we need to discover how to motivate the Arab to be other then he is.

The book has 21 chapters and deals analytically with the psychological makeup of the Arab people. However, there are three chapters which may address the cores of the dysfunctions in Arab culture: **First,** the domination of ruthless rulers who have inflicted enormous pain and suffering on the populace, and who are intoxicated with the pathology of narcissism. The entire energy of the population has to go toward massaging the Egos of these megalomaniacal leaders.

Second, we look at the place of women in Arab society. The female is the container of the honor of the family, and that puts her in a very sensitive position, as she may touch the vulnerability of man. Moreover, the male has the weaker sex (XY) genes, and the male always want to prevail. This is why he often messes up the lives of women. Unfortunately, Arab society has struggled with the issues of women and has subjected them to all sorts of restrictions and sanctions, in the name of protecting them, as if they are little wild children who do not know the right from wrong. This book addresses this concern analytically and hopes to create some awareness in order to free the soul of woman from the bondage of Arab cultural practices.

Third, religion is a big piece of the fabric of Arab society. Arabs are inclined to focus solely on the ritualistic part of religion and ignore the foundations of religion such as faith in the Almighty God. God sent three major religions to the Arab world. The last one was in the person of the Prophet Mohammad (peace be upon Him), to ask the Arabs to be loving and caring human beings, both toward each other, as well as toward the world around them.

Sadly, Arabs have never deeply absorbed the true teachings of God. They are very loud when it comes to talk, but fall short when it comes to practice. Perhaps they have dual personalities or two systems of values that operate opposite each other at the same time. Nevertheless, the Arab individual seems to be living with those two systems of opposing values comfortably, similar to Dr. Jekyll & Mr. Hyde. The soul of the human is comprised of two distinct segments, good and evil. These two separate forces live in continuous and inherent conflict with each other and the world around them.

Moreover, Arabs are struggling with their old Bedouin values such as pride, revenge, aggression, and self-centeredness These stand in conflict with modern human values such as human potential or possibility, common good for others, and justice for all. Perhaps such conflict may never be resolved until there can be a paradigm shift in the collective consciousness of Arab individuals.

In summary, culture in general can have a massive hypnotic effect on people. Persons who are born under certain cultural practices and beliefs tend to act according to the set of roles that the culture has designed for them. In most instances, people are paralyzed by these cultural practices. Their conscious mind can be shackled and they can act like a robot; it can shape their psyche. Thus, I say people are not free as long as the culture indoctrinates them with the blueprint of its agreed upon roles. Whether the culture is Arab or American or Brazilian, all are the same.

Therefore, humanly speaking, we really need to be less judgmental about any cultural practice. Although, some cultures give people some level of freedom within their lives. These cultures have less of a dysfunctional pathology, while the rigid culture, which does not allow people some measure of freedom over their lives, may have more neuroses and dysfunction. That is the core difference when it comes to human behaviors.

In the wisdom of the Tao, wise men do not need to prove their point;
Men who need to prove their point are not wise.

Chapter One

Is There Such A Thing As Arab Psychology?

The science of psychology began with the founding father of experimental psychology, Wilhelm Wundt (1832-1920). Then Sigmund Freud, in the middle of last century, revolutionized the whole concept of the human behavior. These men and others like them offered distinctive perspectives about human behavior by factoring in cultural practices, family upbringing, economic conditions and educational level.

In other words, an individual is born in a specific place in a specific time and under certain circumstances; all of these factors have a tremendous impact on the formation of his psychological makeup. Throughout much of the 20th century, psychology remained embedded in these European and North American patterns of thought.

In recent decades, however, our planet has become more of a "global village". Therefore, many cultures took the science of psychology and tailored it to suit their prevailing values or cultural practices. Carl Jung accentuated the impact of the collective conscience, which mostly is comprised of the cultural practices people inherited from their ancestors.

In answer to the question, "Is there such thing an Arab psychology?" yes, there certainly is, just as there is a Japanese psychology or a Chinese psychology. Each group around the globe: 1) lives in a specific geographic location; 2) shares the same historical struggles; 3) eats certain foods; 4) wears a certain type of clothing; 5) follows the same customs, traditions and cultural practices; 6) speaks a specific language; 7) shares the same religious beliefs; and 8) has a particular educational system. All of these components work collectively to shape the individual psychology for each group, differentiating it from others living elsewhere with a different set of values and cultural practices.

Although there is the above universal principle that shapes behavior in a similar fashion worldwide, it is equally meaningful to conceive of culture as a system that has its own dynamic bounds. These boundaries can create phenomena that appear contradictory to the universal notion of how humans function in their locale, or how their world should be understood by the outsider.

Nevertheless, the psychology of Arabs who lived a hundred years ago was diabolically different from the psychology of Arabs today. It's very similar to saying the people who live in the Amazon region in Brazil are completely different than the people who live in Rio de Janeiro, Brazil. The surrounding environment can shape the psychology of its inhabitants. Thus, there IS a psychology of the Arab, and it is a very complicated one. The tenet of this book is to explore all facets of Arab psychology.

The psychology of the Arab has been shaped by living in the desert; by its shifting sands, which make the Arab temperament volatile. It is shaped by lack of water, causing Arabs to be nomads who move from place to place, to look for water and food for human and animal alike. This is why the Arabs do not have strong alliances to their land; they like to move and immigrate to other places in the world.

The psychology of the Arab has also been shaped by a strong affinity to the tribe to which he belongs. Thus, the concept of nationality is a relative one, because Arabs' alliances must first be to their tribe or community.

It is also worth mentioning that the psychology of the Arab has been shaped by their pompous language, which is very rich in descriptions of their lives in the desert, or their lives under abusive rulers, or their glorious lives in the distant past. Linguists around the world agree that language can sculpt the depth of the psychological structures of people; it is thus with the Arabic language. The Arabic language carved its place in the psyche of the Arab, because it is the language of the holy book, the Quran. English-speaking peoples do not attach to the English language because it is not the language of Christianity. The language of Christianity is Aramaic, the language that Jesus Christ spoke. Aramaic is now spoken by a group of Iraqi Christians called Chaldean.

Moreover, Arab society is a collectivist one, meaning the individual self-concept can be derived from community approval or community acceptance or recognition. It is not the individualistic society as in the West, in which a person derives his own self-concept from his personal merit, or his personal accomplishments and achievements. This factor alone can shape the Arab individual differently from others. Arab culture may be similar to Japanese culture, which also focuses on community. The benefit of society is placed ahead of individual interests.

All these factors collectively characterize the Arab individual and make his psychology unique. The study of the individual within the content of his environment gives a clear picture about his uniqueness. People do not live in isolation; they are surrounded by an environment or culture that influences each reciprocally. There is fluid dynamic interaction among all the cultural factors that make up an Arab psychology, which makes it worthwhile to investigate such a psychology. The purpose is to develop some understanding of why the Arab people behave as they do. Once that is understood by others, they can be less harsh in their judgments, and more compassionate toward Arabs, because they have been through hellish conditions.

Exploring the Arab psychology may give Arabs themselves a fresh looks at their behavior through psychological lenses. In addition, they may try to arm themselves with some courage to change what one might consider neurotic inclinations, which dominate their behavior and make them unhappy people.

Certain views and attitudes can be found in any culture, and these views or attitudes normally characterize people who are living in that culture. If those attitudes are positive or helpful it can color the society with such positivism, as may be seen in Norwegian or Danish society; they have scored very high in the scale of well-being. However, if those views or attitudes are negative then such negativity may become contagious, as we see in Arab society.

Complaints are the prevailing norm in any Arab conversation. You do not see two people getting together without reciting a list of complains over many things in their daily lives. From the poor educational system to poor infrastructure, from lack of sanitation to daily humiliation at the hands of the regime, not to mention the embezzlement of the nation's wealth, Arab culture is infected with many negative elements. Therefore, it is essential to study Arab psychology and shed some light on such psychological phenomena, and therefore help people to have a clear understanding of the causes of Arabs' pain and agony.

Often cultural conditioning allows for the construction of a false sense of self, which may be based on fears. The creative part of the self normally is based on love of life. This is clearly what this book is about: analyzing whether the culture of fear has limited individual possibilities, and manufactured a person who is ruled by neurosis and tyranny.

Chapter Two

The Psychology of Arab Leaders

The Pathology of Narcissistic Personality Disorder

If the country is governed with tolerance,
The people are comfortable and honest.
If the country is governed with repression,
The people are depressed and crafty.
If you want to govern the people,
You must place yourself below them.
If you want to lead the people,
You must learn how to follow them.

Tao Te Ching

For the last hundred years or more, since or even before the Ottoman Empire, the Arab people have suffered from ruthless, despotic and tyrannical leaders. Often, people around the world wonder why Arabs are attracted to such leaders, the majority of whom seem to suffer from some traits of personality disorders. Even Arabs are questioning this trend, which has baffled them for a long time. The trend has cost them an inordinate amount of suffering and agony.

In this analysis, we will try to gain some insights and perspective into such phenomena that have plagued the Arab world for years.

Arab leaders have a grandiose sense of self-importance. Undoubtedly, many of them believe they are essential and indispensable to the survival of their people. For example, Hosni Mubarak said to the people of Egypt, "If I leave the country, it will be in shambles". He has left and the country is functioning well. The other example is Tunisian Ben Ali, who said, "There is no way the people can have a country without me". There is a plethora of examples in this regard.

Moreover, those leaders are preoccupied with the idea that their success with their people can never be duplicated, and would never be seen in other countries. This is a clear case of delusional thinking.

They also see themselves as very powerful. The people around them give them the feeling of omnipotence, as with Saddam Hussein of Iraq. The Iraqis around Saddam made him believe he was so important, that they put his picture everywhere, even on the dishes the Iraqis used.

The leaders also get the feeling that they are brilliant. Saddam once said, "Iraq's infrastructure is far better than any country in the world". Yet, most of the cities in Iraq under Saddam had shortages of electricity, no sewage systems, and lacked clean water. Even so, he governed Iraq for more than 35 years.

Arab leaders are exploitive. They use any means to exploit others, and usually surround themselves with a group of like-minded people. Thus, the people around him tend to feed into his pathology, and he feeds into them. There is reciprocity between the leaders and the people around him, nurturing the dysfunctional behavior of one another. This creates a vicious cycle from which neither is able to break away. This is why the Arab rulers tend to stay in power for such a long time. They surround themselves with a group of people who are in most instances dishonest and who lack a sense of compassion.

Arab leaders require excessive amounts of admiration from their people, surrounding themselves with those who write poetry and songs about how their important leader brought prosperity and good fortune to their people. On the contrary, they brought pain and misfortune to their people. The other part of their psychology is that they think they are special and they are God's gift to the populace. Even when Kasim ruled Iraq in 1960, the masses believed they saw the picture of Kasim in the moon. Of course, that is delusional thinking, and the leaders keep feeding into it.

Moreover, the majority of Arab leaders need a sense of entitlement from their people, to assure the leaders of automatic compliance by the populace. No one questions anything, or raises any objection because the people have to believe that the leader's messages are the law. The leader will say, "I know what is best for the people and I know this is why you must let me rule forever". For example, the president of Yemen changed the constitution to his liking so that he could rule the country for the rest of his life.

Furthermore, the rulers and the people around them are characterized by unbridled greed and the ultimate self-centeredness. Empathy, as in understanding the people's needs, is a very strange concept to these rulers. They have never entertained such thoughts when dealing with their subjects. For example, Gaddafi of Libya described his nation as rats and rodents, while Assad of Syria described his people as "bacteria who do not deserve to live". Even he had no respect for human values.

These rulers are inclined to lack sympathy, and are not willing to recognize the feelings of their people. If anyone might raise his voice or object to what someone has said, that can be considered a grave violation of the dignity of the rulers. This is why the leaders tend to be ruthless and savage when they see any uprising from the people.

They have a strong lust for power and that can blind them from seeing the good for their people.

Being arrogant is one of the characteristics of an Arab leader. They are not 'down to earth' with the populace. However, there was one exception. Sheik Zayid, he may rest in peace, was the last ruler of the United Arab Emirates. He was a special case in that the Arab people remember him with reverence and fondness.

The other personality trait Arab rulers may espouse is that they are very sensitive to any criticism, and even the slightest criticism can be considered a horrific mistake; then that person has to be punished severely. They are impulsive in their decisions and in their reactions to all events. They are not good listeners, nor do they read their history. In addition, they do not learn from their own mistakes or the mistakes of others. Perhaps their grandiosity gets in the way and does not allow them to see the truth of life.

Undoubtedly, they also have some antisocial elements, in which they lie to their people, and have no remorse in their heart with respect to human rights or human dignity. For example, Gaddafi told his people, "I will kill anyone who wants to remove me from my post; and if they insist in doing so I will deliver Libya as a barren place, as I will burn everything to the ground".

As far as the sense of entitlement is concerned, they allow themselves to take or to abuse the wealth of the nation without any accountability. They believe that the wealth is for them and thus do not give any to the people, which is considered theft, rather than just a flaw in their ruling. For example, most of the rulers have stashed huge amounts of money in different investments around the world, and no one can utter any word about it, because this is the right and the privilege of being a ruler and they have no qualms or guilt about it.

Arab rulers are suspicious of others and definitely have paranoid tendencies. At any doubt of someone not being faithful to them, that person will be eliminated from the face of the earth. For example, after the American invasion of Iraq, many mass graves were found. Leaders are preoccupied with conspiracy theories against them. If there is any revolt against them, they tend to blame foreign interventions, because they do not have any insight to reflect on their conduct or how they govern the country. Blame can be used as a defense mechanism to block them from knowing the truth about their nature. If they took a deep look inside themselves, they would know they have to change.

However, the majority of them are not willing even to entertain such thoughts. Insult is part and parcel of their treatment of people around them, and this is why the people who surround these leaders are fearful and cowardly. They are unable to face their leader, so they conform to the letter of the law. Of course, the rulers always want their people to massage their egos; for example, Gaddafi has people meet with him on a monthly basis, and they have to say to him: "you are the greatest of all times". Because of such a dynamic, Arab leaders may live in complete darkness and total ignorance of what is going on in their nation's life.

Shielding themselves from their people is a technique they use to separate/isolate themselves from others, and that is considered having prestige. Transparency is foreign to Arab leaders, and they like to surround themselves with an aura of enigma, with no accessibility. For example, Saddam did not allow even his ministers to meet with him.

As far as Arab leaders' education level, the majority of them are military personnel, and their education mainly consists of Army training. (Kings however are educated and trained in the civilian world.) Thus, other than those who are royalty, these leaders are not educated in human history. Most do not have wisdom in dealing with the challenges they may face with their people. A few of them are even illiterate.

The other inclination, as far as Arab leaders are concerned, is to have inflated, mammoth egos and to feel that people should serve them in any capacity. They are not the servants of their people, as in some parts of the world. In the Arab world, heads of state are self-absorbed with superior attitudes. Thus, there are serious chasms between them and their people. The prevailing view overall is that the people see the rulers as their enemy, and the rulers see the people as their enemy.

In considering trust, Arab leaders often do not trust anyone, even their family members. Therefore, they do not know how to delegate authority and they keep all the power for themselves. For example, people used to have to get Saddam's permission to enroll their children in private school. What a silly thing for a president of a country to be concerned about . . . a child's choice of school!

The other prevailing feeling of Arab leaders is megalomania. Gaddafi has told the media several times that he is the King of the Kings of Africa, and that he is God's gift, sent to the human race. Therefore, if a leader has such a concept of himself, there is no way for him to serve his people. On the contrary, people must serve him with reverence.

When it comes to brutality, Arab leaders have a strong belief that "if you kick the dog often enough, he will either be a coward or vicious". Often they condition people to be cowardly; this is why Arabs stay under such psychopathic leaders for a long time.

On the other side of the equation, the Arab people have been abused for such a long time, they tend to identify with the aggressor. They overvalue their leaders, and feel they have to flatter them to avoid any harm. They must cajole the leaders so they can be safe. In the process of ingratiation and cajoling, people lose their self-trust. More than that, they lose faith in themselves and become angry and aggressive toward each other. As the old wisdom goes, "if you do not trust people, you make them untrustworthy".

Psychologically, the oppressed people have almost as big a need to believe in the legitimacy of the regime that dominates them, as do their oppressors.

Identification with the aggressor can serve psychological purposes; one is to protect oneself from any resulting threat, hostility, and sense of victimhood. Such identification provides the individual a buffering against the fears of vulnerability and sense of being a victim. This psychological identification also works as an incentive for an aggressive outlet, as well as for the desire to victimize others. Therefore, identification serves as a powerful defense mechanism against victimhood.

No doubt, Arab leaders have a serious case of sadistic tendencies. Inflicting pain on their people is a practice they enjoy. Saddam used to watch his gang of thugs throw the opposition's people from a high building. As they reached the ground and their bodies would shatter to pieces, he clapped and laughed.

Arab leaders have mastered the art of manipulation and induce fear in every single member of their society. We know fears produce unintelligent people because they are frozen in their intellect. Literally, Arab people are paralyzed by fear. They are constantly besieged by a multitude of unresolved worries and fears about their lives, jobs, and the futures of their children.

Most of the time Arab leaders are nervous and anxious, because their hearts never know the love for their people. They only know how to abuse and insult people. Because of this treatment, the whole of Arab society has become a society of victims. How can such a society contribute to the human community, other than through aggression and terrorism, because the leaders have planted the seeds of pain and misery in people?

The lust for power is one of the salient characteristics of Arab leaders. Once they obtain office, the first thing they do is eliminate freedom, kill opponents, and begin lying to their people and to the whole world about almost everything. Often they start to believe their own lies. In general, the Arab people are naïve; almost half of the population is illiterate. Moreover, the leaders perpetuate such a status quo. For example, Saddam kept lying to his people that he would defeat the whole world and asked the people to join him. Sadly, they did.

The Arab people are depressed because they face daily humiliation and injustice in their life by their leaders. Once they meet and trust someone, they tend to complain about many things. However, sometimes they are unable to utter a word because they are afraid that person may be an informer to the government. There is a saying among Arab people: "do not say anything, for perhaps the wall has ears to tell on you." Smiling is not a common practice in Arab world. It is said Arabs smile over the injustices dealt them, or over the shortages of food, electricity or water, because the leaders purposely keep people striving after basic survival needs. The leaders in this way prevent the populace from thinking about politics or challenging the government.

There is something unique about Arab leaders in that they are always surrounding themselves with foolish, uneducated advisors. These people generally have low IQs and lack human decency in their hearts. Thus, they tend to give a much-distorted picture about the nation. They often block any flow of real information to the leaders. The Arab people are very aware of such practices, but they have no means to change or challenge it.

Arab leaders consider themselves as the fathers of their nations; thus, people have to exercise absolute unquestioning obedience to them. That can be counterproductive to both the leaders and the people. The people stay immature psychologically because they are treated like children who are told what to do. Moreover, that can also stifle creativity. The leaders themselves also stay immature emotionally because there is no challenge to their authority and consequently they deprive themselves of further emotional or intellectual development. Therefore, Arab leaders are among the least educated leaders in the world, and are the most isolated from what is going on around them in the rest of the world.

We all know there are two forces operating inside each individual. As Freud put it, one is the power of **Eros**, which is the power of love. It is the power of building, helping each other, doing good works for the sake of humanity. This power has contributed greatly in making our world a better place to live. This power has invented all the good technologies to improve the lives of the human race. This power transcends the garbage of selfishness or self-centeredness.

Also inside humans, on the other hand, is the **Thanatos** power, which is the power of death and destruction. It is a primitive power, the power of pure selfishness. This power wages wars, and destroys what we build as the human race. These two powers exist within every individual simultaneously. We struggle daily over which one dominates the other. These powers might also be called the higher self and lower self. The higher self communicates with our benevolent tendencies, while the lower self flirts with the evil forces inside of us, or the dark side of our soul. Some have cultivated their nature and triumphed over the rubbish of the lower self through several means.

The astonishing fact of Arab lives is that the majority of their leaders are operating from the lower self, and have inflicted immeasurable pain and suffering on their people. Either the dark side of their soul is so prevailing they have to control people for the rest of their lives, or they have to destroy the people and the country. For example, Gaddafi indicated clearly, "either I rule people forever or I destroy the country". Mubarek sent his own people to destroy the infrastructure of Egypt.

The latest developments in the Arab world clearly show that those countries' leaders are operating from the dark side of their souls and there is no means to rehabilitate them. Moreover, the Arab people need a serious psychological rehabilitation. This is necessary to undo the incredible damage that has resulted from long years of humiliation, cruelty, lack of freedom, lack of necessities, and most of all, the prevalence of unjust treatment by their leaders. Even though the Arab people are sitting on the richest pieces of land of our planet, with huge deposits of natural resources, they also have the highest unemployment in the world, because the national wealth of the people has been embezzled by their leaders.

Nevertheless, Arab leaders are deficient in social conscience, and are self-indulgent and emotionally detached from their people. They are often callous and disconnected, and have a God complex with a fragile sense of self. They want their people to pander to them with self-glorification. They are vain and contemptuous, emotionally shallow and numb, and they have no capacity for sharing with others unless they benefit from the people around them.

Analytically speaking, Arab rulers have a serious case of the **Ego-syntonic**, which means they abuse people but their conscience never bothers them. They may have delusional disorders or learning disabilities. It appears they may also have arrested personal development, or grow up with an absent or failed father. In addition, the role of a nurturing mother is often not present.

The overwhelming observation here is the Arab leaders are incapable of learning the lessons around them on the world stage. Perhaps that explains their detachment from reality. The world therefore wonders if those leaders are inherently evil, or are they merely a specific phenomenon that infects only the Arab society in this period of history?

In conclusion, the recent developments in Arab world—the revolution of the populace—clearly show that Arab leaders will go to any length to literally destroy the whole country just to stay in power. In other words, it is a very conspicuous example of someone with a syndrome of decay. That is a clear case of antisocial personality, blind malignant narcissism, **or they have a split personality—both parts evil.**

Moreover, historically, Arab rulers of today are no different then the leaders of Omiya Empire or Abbasi Empire or the most recent one, the miserable Ottoman Empire. Those empires ruled the Arab world for a long time, and they were the epitome of corruption and violation of human justice. It is a long history and the true victims are still the Arab people.

Nevertheless, behavioral science has shown us that the anatomy of dictators normally carries the seeds of destruction; first to the people that they rule, and second to themselves. Thus, their demise, without exception, is very shameful.

Chapter Three

The Place of Women in Arab Society

The feminine outlast the masculine
The feminine allows, but the masculine causes
The feminine surrenders, then encompasses and wins

The Tao

In order to understand the Arab's psychology, you must understand the place of the female and the way she has been treated throughout centuries. It is very helpful to go back to review Arab history regarding the attitudes towards women. In the time of **Jaheliah**, this is the time before Islam, Arabs used to feel ashamed of having a baby girl. Thus, they used to bury the girl alive, for two reasons. First, she may bring shame to the family if she is captured and raped by an opponent's tribe. (In Arab tribal society, rivals raided each other.) Second, there was a fear of poverty and the inability to feed them; it was a matter of survival. Arabs throughout centuries suffered from shortages of food and water and one way to survive was to raid another tribe and take their livestock and their water sources. This was the lifestyle of the nomadic Arab. These practices lasted for many centuries until the Prophet Mohammad came (peace be upon Him) and eradicated the practice of burying girls alive and raiding rivals.

Although we know Islam enlightened the Arab, murdering a girl still existed in the subconscious mind of the individual. Even today, the practice of honor killing still exists in limited practice in some parts of Arab world, because Arabs consider women the bearer of their honor. How did they come up with such a concept? Perhaps from medieval society in Europe, when a man put a chastity belt around "his" woman's vagina when he went to war, so she could not cheat on him.

Arabs consider virginity as the pinnacle of their honor. A woman must stay a virgin until she gets married. In some parts of the Arab world the blood from the virginity must be shown to the whole community, as a proof that the bride has maintained and kept intact the honor of the family. Even the business of sewing "virginity" back if the girl lost it has been thriving lately.

Psychologically, virginity represents to a man that he is the first conqueror of a woman, as if he is in battle and the blood represents his victory. Or, he may feel superior to her and have a sense of ownership, because he is the first one to deflower her. Moreover, even today, if a woman has lost her virginity the community tends to frown and look down upon her. Undoubtedly, she may have a hard time finding a spouse because society prefers a virgin to a non-virgin. The male, however, is treated differently; there is no need for him to be a virgin. There is a different yardstick with which to measure him. In fact, the male is more admired if he has conquered many women; people look up to him. He may be considered a very strong man.

This strict adherence to the practice of virginity has kept the Arab woman in an unfavorable place in society. Because she is at the mercy of her conqueror, he has to initiate having her; she cannot take the initiative toward him. This is why Arabs have the highest percentage of spinsters in the world. The Arab world has millions and millions of women who stay at home, waiting for a man to knock on their doors. Often, that man does not come because he is unable to have her and support a family, due to the financial difficulties experienced by a great number of Arab men. If Arab society has a large percentage of the female population who are unmarried, it constitutes serious psychological problems for the whole society. These women feel depression, anger, frustration and disappointment toward their families and the system by which they have been victimized for such a long time.

An Arab woman has no political clout. Her voice is not heard most of the time. She does not have the privileges a man does, and is not taken as seriously as men are. Because of such treatment over time, the Arab woman internalizes her attitudes and she feels inferior to her male counterpart. She even suppresses her femininity and becomes angry at herself and at society in general. Moreover, she reflects such attitudes on her children, and thus Arabs can grow up frustrated because they have a mother who is unhappy with herself. She teaches her children not to express their feelings and even sometimes, she lies to them about the way she feels. Consequently, children pick that up from their mother and become a duplication of her psychology—the psychology of the meek, non-assertive individual.

Society makes her a superficial human being by stripping all of the choices from her life. In some instances, she has no right to choose her life partner. Normally her family may choose for her, while she spends most of her time wandering in the local shopping malls to calm her psychological emptiness and her sadness by merely buying unneeded merchandise.

Undoubtedly, Arabs use religion to justify such practice, but the Islamic religion is far too superior to oppress women. The Prophet Mohammad (peace be upon Him) was the best example of the wonderful treatment of a woman. Nevertheless, the practice of Arabs oppressing women and treating them as handicapped individuals has its historical roots in Jahiliah. It is not easy for the Arab man to give up such practices, which have lasted thousands of years, and have become ingrained in his subconscious mind. For example, if we look to history, the Abbasi Khalifa Almotoical used to have four thousand women—concubines—in his palace (Hitti, History of Arab). Although there has been minor progress for the Arab woman in some areas, equal treatment with the Arab man has not reached the desirable level.

The psychological treatment of Arab women has shaped their personality and caused them to develop **Stockholm syndrome**, which is identification with the aggressor. With any wind of change that may rise up, you will find the first line of attack normally comes from women. This can be a result of an accumulation of years of oppression, which has developed within a woman a negative belief about herself. Furthermore, this has limited her mental creativity and thus, she still walks behind men as far as modern progress is concerned. Women, sadly enough, have bought into such a message and it's becoming a part of their psychological make up, resulting in their prevailing attitude that they are inferior to men.

Psychological wisdom reveals if a person feels inferior, he or she will not live up to their potential and will always be a marginal member of society. This is exactly what has happened to the Arab woman. She has been marginalized and she has conveyed that, directly or indirectly, to her children in the way she has brought them up.

The status of women in Arab society is a very crucial and sensitive subject with which the Arab world has been struggling for a long time. Undoubtedly, this struggle has pulled the society backward and has influenced its development profoundly, not allowing society to move forward.

Arab society is a **patriarchal** one. There is no balance between female and male energy. We know female energy can bring freshness to the equation and make life move smoothly. Females in the Arab world are denied actualizing their full potential, and even if they are assigned to play some roles, they can be minor ones. Consequently, a woman feels not up to her potential and becomes disappointed with herself and with society. No one takes her seriously and then she does not take herself seriously as well. Her role has been concealed even inside of the family. That may make her unable to assume the role of a strong mother who is able to establish or rear a healthy generation with sound self-esteem.

Her self-esteem has been squashed by the attitudes of society and left her an empty shell. As a result of such treatment, Arab society will not participate in any progress unless the woman takes her proper place in society.

There are a myriad of studies clearly indicating that any person who has a strong mother with great self-esteem will grow up healthy psychologically and progress in life with less difficulty. Thus, Arab society will not achieve any degree of development unless it changes its attitudes toward women, and views them as full members with indispensable roles for the greatest good of society.

In contrast, Arab culture also tends to assign unusual power to woman. She is seen as a cunning creature with whom you have to be very aware when dealing. Or she may be considered shrewd; she can take your breath away. She may also be seen as an astute individual who uses her femininity to captivate you and enslave you to her. All of these descriptions are aiming to make her a mysterious being and men need to have all the necessary skills to deal with her. Even with all these skills, men may often fail to please her.

The contradiction in Arab culture is pronounced when men become fearful of female sexuality. This is why the Arab likes to cover the woman from head to toe or put her in total isolation because if she is out on public she may create havoc. This is the prevailing attitude among many people. Arabs like to mask females' identity so they can be absent on the stage of society. This unconsciously indicates that every man is afraid of a woman. However, the irony here is how illogical the cultural yardstick is, that forces the weaker sex, males, to act as the stronger sex. Undoubtedly, such fear may urge him to abuse and control women just to assuage his fear. A man may come up with the argument that he cares and wants to protect women. That is not true; it is just to cover his own fear.

Often an Arab woman exaggerates her love for her children, because she misses the love from her husband or her family. Thus, she has incredible energy toward her children and sometimes this energy may stifle them. Moreover, sometimes she does not allow the umbilical cord to be severed, even if her children get married or move out; the umbilical cord keeps holding them to her. Of course, that does not make them independent individuals and may also deprive them of personal maturity.

An Arab woman may live with her husband for many years and she may tell him that she loves him. In reality, she does not love him, because she had no choice to marry or divorce him in the first place. She is limited in her choices in many areas of her life, thus she is inclined to camouflage her own real feelings and emotion. She does not present her real self and tends to compromise in most instances, in order to survive in a society that so limit her options.

In general, she lives in constant fear because she does not know when her husband might come home with another woman. Arab culture is a **polygamist** one. Thus, she is insecure and anxious most of the time.

We also have to understand the psychology of woman in a larger scope: that the aim of being loved is stressed more than the aim of loving. A woman may have strong narcissistic needs and the dependency on another object of her love is greater. This is why we see her compensating the missing love in her life by being so loving to her children.

Undoubtedly, there is imbalance in the structure of Arab society between the roles of women and the roles of men. In fact, there is a theory that an Arab man fears that a woman may castrate him, because he is unsure of his own sexuality. Therefore, he has to oppress her. One of the manifestations of the fears that characterize Arab men is the cry over virginity and honor.

Perhaps the phenomenon of oppressing women is not a strange concept to many societies in the history of humanity. Normally the oppressor is the male who feels that woman has the most precious and powerful organ (the vagina), which he considers the seat of pleasure that man seeks all of his life. Once she captivates him, he strives to free himself from the overwhelming desire to go back to the vagina. He feels helpless and weak in the face of his sexual desire. Thus, he oppresses and controls a woman as a defense mechanism, to cool his anxiety.

The question presents itself: why do Arab men oppress and fear women? The analytical psychology states man in general has oppressed woman. But why are the fear and oppression more pronounced in Arab culture?

Simply, males in the Arab culture are not allowed to mature as independent individuals. The male is not given the opportunity to actualize his potential as a useful human being. He, too, is oppressed and marginalized. Thus, he has to displace his anger and frustration on another segment of society, and the weakest link is women.

We all know in behavioral science that a strong, self-assured man will not abuse a female member of his society. However, it is a sad fact that men in the Arab world face enormous hostility by the rules, by the tribal system, or even by a dictatorial father. Thus, he feels helpless and weak. Therefore, he has to take it out on someone else, normally a woman. Perhaps that is the root of the psychological dysfunction in the Arab world, which has led to a cycle of frustration and disappointment in each other. Men are unable to fulfill their innermost desires and thus project their own weakness and insecurity on women. That can clearly be seen in psychotherapy when we are faced with angry and hostile couples. Hence, the course of therapy in such instances is to make them aware of their innermost insecurity and disappointment.

On the other hand, we as males may regress to our early years of life when we were afraid of our mother. Or we may model after our father when we see him mistreating our mother so we mistreat women in general. It is this family dynamic which brings itself into play on the stage of the subconscious mind.

Chapter Four

Learning Helplessness in Arab Lives

There were landmark studies in 1967 by Martin, Seligman and Maier about human behaviors and how circumstances shape people's attitudes, and push them to be helpless and hopeless. The first experiment was conducted with two groups of dogs; one group was placed in harnesses so they could not escape, while the other group was left free with no harnesses. Both groups were then presented with small electric shocks. After this, they placed both groups again in a shuttle box.

A distinct difference was observed between the dogs who had been harnessed and those who had not. The dogs that were unharnessed, when shocked, tried different methods to escape, and jumped across the barrier to avoid the uncomfortable shock. The previously harnessed dogs showed distress, (as did the other dogs), but this group failed to escape the shocks and ultimately lay down on the grid and whimpered. Those dogs harnessed in the first box were not harnessed in the second box, but they submitted to the condition and never even jumped to run away from the shocks; they learned the attitude of helplessness. Humans are like dogs in this way; under particular circumstances they learn to be helpless.

The other study was about frogs. Normally, we know frogs jump if they are put in any uncomfortable situation. The subject frogs were placed in heated water and they jumped right away.

The same frogs were then put in cool water, and slowly the water was heated. Over time, the frogs died from the heat, as if they could not feel the gradual increase, and they were unable to jump. Often humans are like frogs in that we are heated up to our own destruction and learned that there is no exit from our helpless condition. That is exactly what has transpired in the lives of the Arab people.

These studies demonstrated that human beings can be like animals and learn to behave passively or even become paralyzed with inaction if they are faced with painful circumstances. The Arabs have been faced with a lot of suppression and brutality; thus, they learned the attitude of being helpless and meek. The Arab culture has been imbued with the colors of oppression and violation of its people for a long time.

The human condition clearly shows that if we witness a failure either in ourselves or in others, then the less likely we are to attempt change, even if the circumstances change drastically. Hence people perceive events as uncontrollable and unpredictable, and consequently experience more stress and less hope about making a change in their lives.

The American sociologist Harrison has suggested that learning helplessness goes beyond individual psychology, into the realm of social action. When a culture or political identity fails to achieve desired goals, then the perception of collective ability will suffer.

Another way of learning behavior and attitudes is through vicarious learning or modeling. People learn helplessness by observing others who encounter uncontrollable events or circumstances.

These experiments by Seligman and other behavioral scientists have laid the foundations suggesting that human behavior and attitudes, or even beliefs, can be engineered and shaped through systematic reinforcement of the same.

As far as Arabs are concerned, they have been subjugated to many "electric shocks", metaphorically speaking. Like those dogs in the Seligman experiment, or the frogs in the heated bathtub, they have been ruled by despots and tyrannical leaders who literally oppress them for a long time, moving the people to develop a negative view of themselves and others. If an individual develops these feelings, he will be crippled psychologically and unable to move society forward. That explains the backwardness of Arab society.

The Arab has been living under systematic deprivation of their basic individual freedoms or choices. Therefore, they have learned that uttering any word may have detrimental consequences on their well-being. In most instances, they lose their livelihood or even their lives. Often if an individual opposes or objects to the rules in the Arab world, he will be expelled from his job; there will be no opportunity for him to support himself or his family financially. It is a very drastic measure to quiet people's voices.

The psychological picture of the Arab population clearly shows that the average Arab suffers from chronic anxiety, depression, obsessive thinking and somatic complaints, because there is no outlet for their frustration with their conditions. Overall, they are treated with disrespect and without dignity, and therefore develop **self-loathing** attitudes.

The Arab society is not a happy one, because the components of happiness are social equality, control over one's life and freedom of expression. These are non-existent, even though they constitute the "magic triangle" of well-being in any society. Robert Sapolsky observed a group of baboons that lost their control to the Alpha male; they became distressed and suffered many physical illnesses.

At the human level, a form of subordination can influence long-term physical health. Take, for example, the citizens of East Germany when they lived under state power, which was widely feared. They expressed their feelings of helplessness through absent smiles on their faces, according to the research that was conducted by Gabriele Oettingen. Even their self-confidence was less then their West German counterparts. Moreover, there is a statistical relationship between life expectancy and social inequality. Life expectancy among Arab individuals is less then in the West, maybe around 67 years.

The key to individual well-being is the control over one's own life, because losing one's autonomy can be a devastating experience. Arabs suffer from a serious loss of their autonomy, because Arab society is collectivist, in which the individual builds up his own self-concept through the approval of the community. Western society, by contrast, is individualistic, which means the individual develops his self-concept through his own merits and personal accomplishments. In a collectivist society, people around you may interfere in your autonomy and one loses his independence. However, this is not always the case. For instance, Japanese society is collectivist, but there is a great respect for individual choice. The Arab culture is totally a different case, and the makeup of their psychology may accentuate the roles of the father or the elders.

Because of feeling helpless, Arab individuals are less likely to trust one another, let alone trust their rulers. This attitude creates serious trouble for the whole society because there is no trust. Sometimes even family members do not trust each other, because they fear someone may inform on them to the rulers. This results in weak social ties in Arab society, which makes corruption easier to thrive. The worst example of that is what happened in Iraqi and Syrian society. Those two states were run by the secret police, making people feel truly worthless.

Arab society has been plagued by corruption, mismanagement and a chaotic relationship between rulers and people. None of them is working for the common good of society, because people are always inspired to fulfill their individual possibilities. While that can be a great disappointment in the Arab world, this is why most of the "intelligentsia" of the Arab world immigrates to other parts of the world to fulfill their possibilities.

In most instances, the Arab individual feels there is no exit from his own misery, just like the harnessed dogs. This is primarily why the Arab has not contributed to the progress of the human community; they feel helpless and hopeless and are preoccupied solely with their own unfortunate circumstances. There is no energy left to even think about the well-being of others, if well-being has been confiscated. Simply, a depressed person has no interest in the world around him.

Arabs are therefore unable to relate to the world, and often have hostility toward the world in general, because they are envious. Why do other countries have such decent rulers while Arabs have abusive ones? If an outsider observes two Arab individuals conversing, the whole conversation is normally a citation of complaints over everything: the high price of rice, traffic jams, poor infrastructure, lack of free thought, favoritism, nepotism, and moreover the imbedded corruption in the fabric of society. Milgram indicates that most people can bring themselves to behave sadistically under the influence of authority. Feeling helpless and hopeless is a predisposing factor to act as with violence. This is why Arabs behave this way.

Neurologically speaking, the Arab brain has depleted all the serotonin and worries have absorbed all the dopamine; thus, the Arab brain is running on empty. Arabs worry over their daily survival, worry over their children's future and worry over their well-being under ruthless rulers who have induced fears within every single cell of the Arab brain.

Finally, as Erich Fromm put it so elegantly in his book *To Have or to Be:* "when people learn the dynamic of helplessness; they are inclined to become sheep, lose their faculty for critical thinking, feel powerless, and are passive." People who live under a corrupt political system and tyrannical social orders are less creative, less inventive, less assertive and unable to move away from their selfish nature. When this happens in any society, it creates a society of people who literally have no soul.

Chapter Five

The Psychology of Arab Religion

Idol Worship

Throughout history, since the time of the prophet Abraham, Arabs have worshipped idols. They have sculpted a piece of stone, designated a magical power to it, and then put in their homes to worship it, and called it God. This practice continues to the present.

Almighty God has sent several prophets to warn and advise Arabs to worship God, the creator of this universe, instead of worshipping stones. The last Prophet to come was Mohammad [peace be upon Him], who came and asked the people to believe in the Almighty God. Initially they resisted him strongly, fought him hard and refused to leave their long years of idol worship. Eventually, after many years of struggle that the Prophet Mohammad endured, they changed and started to believe in God.

Hence, we may look to the modern Arab and ask, did they really change or are they still worshiping idols? The painful answer is yes, they still worship idols, but in different forms and shapes. Rather than worshiping stones, today they worship personalities, either the head of the government, the head of the tribe, or even the head of the house. The long years of worshiping stones have carved their pathway in the Arab's unconscious mind. It is not easy to erase that practice completely; therefore, they have replaced it with **the cult of personality**.

Arabs are inclined to idealize their leaders, the head of their community or even the head of the office where they work. Often the place of work has an idol. Undoubtedly, the person who is being idolized loves it and gradually starts to have an inflated ego. The consequences of such a practice are very detrimental to the whole society, because in doing so we are indirectly training or creating persons who can be despots, and those despots eventually will subjugate the whole society to unbearable abuses.

The excessive admiration and glorifying of leaders, fathers, tribal elders, or the heads of government is just a replacement form of worshiping stones. Perhaps, if the Arabs had continued to just worship stones, it would have been far better for us as a society. Stones do not have inflated egos and the power to abuse people, while modern idols never hesitate to abuse and inflict tremendous pain and suffering on the people (there are several examples, such as Ben Ali of Tunisia, Assad of Syria, Ghadafi of Libya or Mubarak of Egypt).

Arabs are tormented about religion and they carry serious conflicts within their hidden selves, because the strong **Superego** tends to run into severe conflict with the **Id.** For example, an individual may preach morality, but is not following it in his daily life. For instance, he may drink alcohol but preach abstinence from alcohol. In psychological terminology, this is called **compartmentalization,** which means once can be moral in one instance and immoral in another. Internally, an individual may see nothing wrong with such behavior, nor does it cross their mind to think otherwise.

Arabs are pleasure seekers. They are hungry for spiritual pleasure, and thus they adhere to the ritualistic practices of religion so they can derive some pleasure, as there is a relationship between pleasure and belief. Perhaps, the pleasure of controlling others is more pronounced through religion, and so religion in the Arab world can be used as a form of control. That control results in the subjugation of others. That in itself may be a form of satisfaction to an ego hungry for control. Often the majority may also use religion to persecute others, or advance his own personal interest. In such cases, the fear of hell or love of heaven is secondary to him.

We know that the three most dominant religions, Judaism, Christianity and Islam, all spring from the Arab world. Perhaps, God knew that the Arab was living in total darkness and sent His messengers to salvage the Arab's soul from evil forces. So while Arabs have laid the moral laws for the world, they are the first ones to delight in breaking the rules of these great religions.

The relationship between Arabs and religion can be a very complex one. The individual tends to carry the seeds of contradictions. For example, he may pray five times a day and read the Holy book, but his behavior is dysfunctional and he does not hesitate to violate the simple rules of ethics. Contradictions are one of the most salient features of the Arab personality. Moreover, the Arab personality has two faces, the outer face and the inner face, or the public face and the private face. Often, the private face does not correspond with the public face. Thus, he may live his entire life with two faces or more. The public face is for show and social acceptance; the private face is his real self. The Arab thus has some superficial tendencies that surface to negotiate living in society.

Arabs are the least people to follow the rules of religion, because the great religions have organized our lives and defined the laws that govern our behaviors. For example, religion clearly shows us how to be honest and sincere in our jobs; Arabs are very disrespectful of their jobs and they do not have regard for time. Moreover, they do not have a desire for completion of a task.

The majority of Arabs are not spiritual beings. They do not know this sophisticated concept. They are Bedouins and they know how to take advantage of each other. These are the values of the desert. It is very difficult for them to comprehend the real values of religion, because they still struggle with basic survival needs. They cannot adhere to lofty concepts of religion while their stomachs are growling.

Arabs have benefited psychologically from the great religions, in that they have a strong belief in the concept of fate, which is that everything is predetermined by God. That has helped the Arab greatly by alleviating pain and suffering.

The purpose of the instruction of religion is to counter the selfish, greedy, mediocre nature of man. Unfortunately, Arabs still have a long way to go to adapt to the true teaching of religion. One may apply that statement to the majority of people on our planet. However, Arabs are exceptional for being defiant to the teaching of religion, because the values of the desert tend to supersede any other values. The harshness of their environment has shaped the psychological tendency to be cruel to each other.

There are three components to every religion: **faith, conduct/ behavior and rituals**. We know faith is the most important component of any religion. The second in the hierarchy is conduct and the third is ritual. Most of the people around the world have maintained the practice of rituals. There are great resources and wealth still pouring into building places for practicing rituals. Undoubtedly, that can be at the expense of faith and conduct.

Arabs are wonderful in practicing religious rituals, but as far as faith is concerned, it can be far from their reality. They spend an inordinate amount of time in rituals performance. More importantly, the core of their faith can be disconnected from the real lives of people. The psychological explanation is that the Arab individual feels that practicing religious rituals can substitute for faith, because this is what he wants to show people. Only God can see faith. He is more concerned about what others may see of him. In our collectivist society, we care about other's opinions of us, while faith is a very private matter and only God knows what is in our hearts.

One of the main principles of religion is the principle of justice for all. Sadly, this principle in particular is almost absent from the lives of Arabs, from the nuclear family to the governmental level.

The religious lives of Arabs can serve as a reaction; a defense mechanism Arabs use when they are overwhelmed with inner anxiety. It is the presentation of the opposite of the individual's inner desires. For example, a person may be very loud and vehement in public about honesty and virtuosity, while in private he is very dishonest and deceitful. This person is trying to assuage his anxiety over being deceitful by trying to be loud about something that is very different from what he has inside himself. Arab individuals collectively are using such defense mechanisms to manage their internal conflict.

In conclusion, we teach people religion, we also pay much attention to ritualistic behavior, but we do not teach people responsibility and respect toward their fellow human beings, which is the core of religion. However, the Transparency International Organization considers Arabs one of the most corrupt societies on the planet. So, what is the outcome of all this teaching? The answer is very clear: the Arab's focus on rituals, not on the core faith. Clearly, the Holy book indicates that the most important aspect of religion is complete faith in the teaching of Almighty God.

One of the landmarks of Islamic teaching is justice for all. However, we see almost a conspiracy of silence. People see the missing justice, the corruption and the cruelty, but they do not say anything about it. They are fed up, assuming there is no point in speaking out. The whole situation is very overwhelming.

Chapter Six

Arab Thinking Processes

Any culture may imbue and shape its citizens with certain thinking processes. Arabs are characterized by pre-logical thinking and magical thinking, meaning one can master what can name. For example, if I am upset at you and I threaten you by saying, "I will burn your house", merely saying it is enough to fulfill me psychologically with no need to carry out the action. One can master what one can name. Words can be a substitute for action.

Perhaps that can be attributed to the tyranny of the social and political system. The individual feels impotent, thus he can only use words, with inability to carry out the action. When an outsider hears the pompous words of an Arab they may wonder, "Is it true, what they are saying?" Of course the answer is no, just the magic of saying the words gives the person psychological satisfaction. The omnipotence of words is embedded in the Arab thinking processes.

On the other hand, Arabs are inclined to overemphasize the significance of words and pay less regard to actions. That can be also a result of the psychological replacement of actions by words. For example, if someone talks about virtue, he sees himself as a virtuous person yet he does not need to follow that with action. The entire culture focuses on words, thus it is considered a verbal culture. Moreover, you have to win the verbal battle if ever faced with it.

Such thinking can be archaic, and possibly, it emerged from the unpleasant reality that individuals cannot influence action. So by saying something, that gives false empowerment.

Often Arabs are excellent in voluntarily giving advice on any subject. That may bring them some happiness, because they feel they mastered what they just said. The other characteristic of Arab thinking is the shift from one topic to another; you may observe incoherency in the thinking process. Arabs have not been trained in logical thinking, because school curriculums are poor when it comes to the process of thinking. Moreover, the pressure from society can be overwhelming, and thus the individual is unable to be unique or clear in his thinking, because of the fear of judgment by others. This stands in the way of any free logical development. For example, if a poet writes poetry which is not understood by the public that may add a mystical quality to his writing. The fact that the public does not understand it can be in his favor.

Fear of judgment by others can be a nightmare in the Arab thinking process. Individuals always need to take what others may think of them into consideration. As I indicated in another chapter of the book, Arab society is a collectivist culture, which means individuals develop their self-concepts through others' perception. Thus, individual thinking may become a hostage to the community's judgment and social approval. The message is clear: if you do not follow society's way of thinking, you will be castigated and ostracized.

Arab thinking is group thinking, and those groups always live within huge walls surrounding most cities of the Arab world. This has influenced their thinking profoundly. Most of time Arab thinking is within the wall/box of their societies. Interestingly, the psychological translation of the actual wall that surrounds Arab cities is the wall around Arab thinking. The thinking comes out of the wall that the culture has constructed for them.

The other thinking process that the Arab is inclined to have is the preoccupation with sexuality. As we know there is clear segregation between males and females in the Arab world.

(Modern Arab societies are less restricted to such segregation.) Thus, Arab individuals stay curious about the opposite sex. Sexual thinking can consume a lot of energy; they even write or recite poetry over the woman missing from the equation. Although, in Arab private daily lives, sexual conversations can dominant all other conversation.

Throughout history, Arabs have been traders. Thus, their way of thinking is inclined to be in terms of benefits and losses. That may be reflected in how they deal with each other. The message here is clear: if I do not benefit from you then there is no use for you, to me. That can be seen in friendship practices and other daily transactions. The whole society has adapted utilitarian attitudes.

In this way of thinking, society does not normally progress toward a common good of the people. However, there are certain noble ideas that transcend the gain/loss or worth basis of thinking, and make Arabs more human. Unfortunately though, there is no civic sense in Arab society; everyone is looking after their own personal gains and in the process undoubtedly steps over the weak and unfortunate segments of society. This is why there are many downtrodden people in the Arab world.

Another aspect of Arab thinking is immaturity. There are unwritten rules by which each individual is evaluated and accepted according to three hidden criteria. First, if you come from an influential family, you have a place in society; second, if you come from a rich family, you are valued and appreciated; third, if you come from a powerful government position, you are feared and respected. According to these malicious criteria, if an Arab individual does not belong to one of these categories, he is a marginalized human being and his place in society is unnoticed and ignored.

Undoubtedly, the majority of people in Arab society do not belong to any of these groups. Thus, they suffer from neglect and lack of appreciation. These segments of Arab society often suffer from depression, humiliation, and unheard voices. You may find such groups of society are also infected with poverty, lack of education and a high crime rate.

Such thinking processes make a large portion of the Arab population discounted as active meaningful members of their community. Because of the above criteria, those people carry within themselves the seeds of disappointment and chronic discontent. All these contributing factors influence the thinking process and make Arab society an unhealthy one. Moreover, breeding discontent is the landmark of young peoples' thinking in the Arab world.

Finally, the thinking process of powerless people invites two things: first, try to please those on whom they are dependent, and second, attempt to be as much like those in power as possible. They may idealize people in power, and that definitely will lead to self-hate. Hence, a vicious cycle cripples the process of Arab thinking and makes Arabs non-inventive or uncreative people. Overall, the element of fear predominantly colors Arab thinking.

Chapter Seven

Factors That Influence the Psychology of the Arab

B.F. Skinner was a prominent behavioral psychologist and a pioneer in studying the influence of the environment on the individual. Arab people are no different than the rest of humanity in that they have environmental factors which profoundly shape their psychology, in spite of conscious desires. We may summarize the following factors:

1. *The Educational System.* The educational system in the Arab world is based on memorization, and primarily on verbal memorization. Children in school may memorize the whole poems, or long speeches of important Arab icons. The system does not, and has never allowed, critical thinking to occur or develop.

    From elementary school through college, the whole foundation of education is that the subject presented to students must be memorized. When examination time comes, they "pour out" their knowledge on paper to get good grades; that is all that counts. Moreover, most of the subjects are not related to the lives of the individual. Thus, when people come to the job market they do not have practical knowledge to apply in the real world.

They therefore become frustrated and disenchanted with the whole process of employment. Or, they may be faced with favoritism in the hiring process. To a large degree, employment in the Arab world is based on who you know, not on personal merit.

The other characteristic of the educational system is control. There is no open communication between students and teachers; rather, there is a gap, because the teacher considers himself as the person who renders knowledge and the students should be the container of this knowledge. Moreover, they train students to accept the knowledge imparted wholesale without any input from the students themselves.

The Arab educational system never tackles the curiosity of students. Therefore, school can often be a boring place for students and they do not wish to be there. The educational system never addresses the needs of society or the personal needs of the students, never taking into consideration their stages of development.

Sadly, personal development is seen as a waste of time, because the reward after graduation is often unemployment. This is why Arabs have the world's highest rate of unemployment among college graduates. For example, they may need one hundred teachers to teach the Arabic language in a country, but three thousand teachers of Arabic graduate and every day they go to the ministry of education to ask for employment. Of course, they are turned away, and told there will be no jobs for Arabic language teachers for the next ten years.

So the irony is, those teachers who graduated from an Arabic language program may apply to work in banks or other places not related to their training. Then they may need training in the banking (or other) system. The new employee becomes frustrated, because they are cognitively inclined to teach Arabic. This is what they have been trained for, yet they have to shift mentally to banking. Consequently, they may do a poor job in the bank, because they took the job to have a livelihood, not out of an interest in the banking system. Thus, when you go to the bank in the Arab world, you may find a large number of frustrated employees.

The education system in the Arab world is also archaic. It was introduced at the time of colonization in the middle of the last century, and still the schools operate from this same concept.

The educational system in Arab world has contributed greatly to keep the Arab world backward technologically. They do not encourage or establish experimentation to open the mind of the individual. Moreover, the educational system also has contributed to solidify the position of the rulers. Students learn that their opinions do not matter, and the best thing that can happen to them is to have such rulers.

This educational system does not spend money on research, thus there are no scientific endeavors. Teachers do not even update themselves with the latest knowledge in their field. They think, "What is the point? Whether you are earnest or fake, it is the same." There is no clear system of reward in the schools. It all depends on who you know. Giving favor is quite common in the Arab world.

The other troubling factor in education is the use of the English language and the inferiority of using Arabic. No human development can take place in any society unless people can use their native language. Arabs in general are not proud of their language, and see themselves inferior. Once this concept takes place in their collective consciousness there is serious trouble with their national development.

2. *Illiteracy.* The illiteracy rate in the Arab world is high. It may reach more than 50% in some countries, and this percentage may even be higher among rural areas and higher yet among females. For instance, in Yemen more than 80% of women do not read or write. As these illiterate women raise children, no doubt the children may suffer

from many dysfunctions. Of course, the percentage varies from country to country.

3. *Poverty*. Arab populations are sitting on great wealth and they have abundant natural resources, but their wealth has been squandered by their rulers and the elite class in society. The average Arab lives at or below the poverty level. Life for them is a constant struggle to secure the future of their children. The rate of unemployment is very high among young Arabs, with as many as 40% of young people unemployed in some countries. This situation presents a serious problem for the government of these countries. They face unrest constantly, such as what has transpired lately in the Arab world.

4. *Tribal affiliation*. Tribal affiliation can be a hindrance to the souls of people, because their alliance is not to their country or to the good of their community; it is to the tribe. Even educated people still have these attitudes. This affiliation keeps Arabs at a primitive level of kinship. The humanistic/modern view of the universe is that we all are the children of a loving God, and we have to relate to each other from the human level, rather than from the narrow perspective of the tribe. The more education a society has, the less likely it is to identify with tribal values. The eastern part of the Arab world is still involved in the tribal system, while the western part of Arab world (like Morocco) is moving away from it.

5. *Male domination*. The Arab society is a patriarchal society. The role of the male is dominant, and that has tipped the balance of energy in the society. Psychologically, it is very healthy to maintain a co-educational system that stimulates children to compete and excel in their educational endeavors. Man and woman have worked together side by side in the field since creation. If we segregate them, it can create many problems, particularly when we accentuate the roles of male over female. Then social balance will be crippled, which has negative consequences on the whole of society.

Humans are created to be together, and we have desire to be with each other. When we segregate genders, there can be dire consequences, which can threaten the fabric of society, such as anger, frustration, distortions of reality, apathy, and lack of motivation to do the right thing.

6. *Female castration*. The female in the Arab world is marginalized and often she plays a minor role in society. Because honor is attached to her, she is treated with suspicion and mistrust. These attitudes have shaped the concept of society and affected her place in the family. If a woman has a low self-concept, then she may render that to her children. Thus, a child growing up in such a home will be dependent and non-assertive, with a poor self-image. Undoubtedly, this societal orientation has influenced the Arab society and caused it to lag behind the progress of the human community.

7. *The Bedouin mentality*. The other contributing factor shaping the Arab psychology is the nomadic mentality. This can be characterized by self-centeredness, selfishness and harshness, with no affinity to land or nation. This mentality takes advantage of others, and demands complete adherence to the hierarchical system in society. And normally, in such systems the power of the dagger settles disputes.

8. *The Wasta practice or favoritism*. This practice, which means some individuals get favor in gaining something over other people, has prevailed in the Arab world for a long time,. Normally persons who have connections tend to get ahead in many areas in their lives. For example if you know people, you maybe admitted to college even if you have low scores, while the person with high scores may be unable to get in because he/she does not have connections. Or, someone may get his driver's license even if he does not know the basic roles of driving, because, he may use people to help him get it.

There are a myriad of examples that put certain people in places of advantage, and put others at a disadvantage.

Undoubtedly, this is part of the corruption in the Arab world and is endemic. There is no fair or equal treatment of people. Therefore, persons in the Arab world are disappointed and they do not have loyalty to their country.

Transparent International Organization ranked the Arab world as the lowest on the ladder as far as corruption. Corruption has touched every aspect of Arab lives. Psychologically, that can demoralize people; make them angry, frustrated and non-productive. The unfair treatment and injustice that they face in their daily lives gives their reality a bitter taste, and makes them run away even from their skin, so to speak.

All these factors collectively have played significant roles in molding the psychology of the Arab, making them the way they are. Thus, we may ask people from other societies to be less judgmental about the Arabs, and try to understand why Arabs act the way they do. Almost every facet of Arab society has conspired to produce individuals who are basically shy, non-assertive, angry, frustrated, and compliant, having dual personalities with a troubling self-image.

Chapter Eight

The Psychology of the Desert Inhabitants

There are much scientific researches indicating a serious, profound impact of nature or surroundings on human behavior. **Ibn Khaldoun**, an Arab scholar, wrote thoroughly about this subject in his book, *Mugaddimah*. Human beings interact with nature every single minute of their lives. Thus, nature can shape an individual's characteristics. For example, if nature or the environment is generous (e.g., it has an abundance of water and trees), then those who live in such surroundings may become giving beings. If nature or the environment has a lot of rain and trees, it can have a positive impact on a person. If nature is a desert and has nothing to give except sand and rocks, it may make people less giving, or they can be harsh and less generous because they reflect what nature offers them.

If we observe the inhabitants of our planet, Earth, we can clearly see the influence geography has on human beings. For example, people who live close to the water tend to be more relaxed than people who live in the desert. Or, people who live in very lush, green surroundings tend to be accommodating individuals, while those who live in the desert are less accommodating and self-absorbed. This can explain why Arabs are not a relaxed people. They tend to be agitated and self-centered because they have been living for thousands of years in a harsh desert among sand, rocks, and dry wind. Moreover, the desert has limited resources, and it is stingy and hostile toward its inhabitants. Even though in modern times Arabs have accumulated great wealth, the image of the scarcity of the desert still haunts them. And, the poverty of the environment has translated to poverty in their thinking. As a result, the environment has shaped the psychology of Arab people.

The punishment of the desert has a profound impact on the personality of the Arab individual and has imbued them with certain characteristics. For example, they tend to be difficult to deal with, suspicious of others, and greedy because living in the desert is very difficult; they have no control over shifting sand or availability of water. We, as human beings, tend to inherit certain traits in our personalities. The subjugation of living in a harsh environment, one that shows no mercy, for many centuries can make us a hostile people. Similarly, Eskimos who live in a land that has been covered with ice for thousands of years tend to be difficult people. Such a lifestyle may prevent individuals from becoming innovative people.

According to Abraham Maslow's hierarchy of needs, people must first satisfy their basic needs such as the need for food, water, and shelter. Then they can move to the second level of need fulfillment, the need for safety and security.

The Arabs have lived for thousands of years in an empty desert, struggling to meet their basic survival needs: the need for food, water, and shelter—although, the tent has not protected them from the dusty wind. This, then, is sufficient reason for their anxiety over what the next day might bring them.

People often suffer from hunger and thirst and act accordingly. Arabs have not felt safe and secure in the desert since tribes often raid one another and took the water or the camel from each other to satisfy their own hunger or thirst. Therefore, attacking each other was a matter of survival, and taking another's livestock was a normal way to survive.

The third level of need fulfillment is the need to be loved. As human beings we need to feel the sense of warmth being loved provides. Arabs, unfortunately, have not reached this third stage in the hierarchy of need fulfillment. They have continued to struggle with the first and second stages: having food and shelter and having their families and themselves safe and secure from harmful attack.

As a result of the severe influence the desert has on the Arab personality, we can clearly see how certain characteristics developed. For example, Arabs generally lack freedom of expression as well as a sense of wholeness in either themselves or each other.

A basic concept in the science of human behavior tells us that people who struggle with their survival needs tend to have difficulty achieving self-actualization or spiritual connections with other human beings. Even though Arabs are now living a modern lifestyle, the accumulation of thousands of years of hardships remains in their collective consciousness. This is the archetype of which Carl Jung talks, that which we inherit from our ancestors.

Moreover, life in the desert deprives the Arab of living creatively or realizing their personal potential. The focus has been on self and on what could be acquired for day-to-day survival. Thus, the selfish nature of the Bedouin is the operating norm of the Arab's daily life. The nomadic Arab tribes moved around, following the water for grazing and for their survival. As a result, they have not developed an attachment to a land or a country, in other words, there is no loyalty for their country, and their daily behavior is the best proof of that. Their own personal gain is the primary motive for their behavior, with a resulting serious disregard for the well-being or the welfare of others. These are common attitudes of the Arab's daily lifestyle, and that was why God sent the Prophet Mohammad (peace be upon Him) to cultivate the cruel nature of most of the Arab. But, it seems the beautiful teaching of Islam has not changed them fundamentally.

Nature surrounding the Arab is static and is the same in whatever direction they turn their face. This may produce boredom within the individual. On the contrary, people who live in season changing surroundings tend to experience pleasurable meaning in their lives; there is no consistent routine in their life as there is in the desert life. The abundances of water tend to produce a soothing effect upon people, evoking a sense of renewal of life and strength. The best example of such an effect occurs in the city of Curitiba, Brazil, of which 75% is green. According to an environmental report, the inhabitants of the city are very positive people, and the city is considered to be the best place in the world to live.

Sadly enough, the Arab are pouring a lot of concrete and cement in their city as insecure reaction to the tent life-style which they have lived for thousands of years. Thus, it is imperative that they invest their wealth in making their land green. Nevertheless, the painful fact remains, even now, Arabs are haunted by an inherent psychological insecurity. We have to look for the applicable solution to the predicaments that face the Arab and understand how their collective conscious mind works. The new generation of Arabs might remove some of the residues of the long-lasting effects of the desert lifestyle. In the meantime, they must transcend over their hostile situation, and free their souls from the punishment of their environment.

Chapter Nine

The Psychological Makeup of Arab Society

Some Common Cultural Practices

Culture consists in the sum total of efforts we make to avoid being unhappy.
Defense systems against anxiety are the stuff that it is made of culture.

Geza Rohein

Generosity. One of the landmarks of the Arab culture is being generous. That can be manifested in feeding others. Arabs like to feed others well and show them that they are very generous people. This cultural practice has historical roots, as Arabs mostly were inhabitants of the desert. Normally a desert has limited resources, thus the best thing that a host can offer guests when they are stranded in the desert, is food. As there were no restaurants at that time, people were obliged to accommodate each other, even though there was a shortage of food, because nothing can grow in the desert. Thus, feeding or giving to others was considered the ultimate generosity, and still is today. It is a very old tradition in Arab lives, and today if you visit an Arab home, they will offer you what they have. Even though they may have very limited resources, Arabs extend themselves and go beyond their means just to show their hospitality.

Undoubtedly that will give the host some psychological satisfaction and will thus give him an edge over others. Food has played a pivotal role in Arab lives, thus, offering food to visitors means that the giver wants to nurture the recipient. Is that not what mothers do, when they love their children . . . give them food?

Cooking. Another skill Arabs have is the art of cooking. Food as a commodity is very valuable in Arab lives, thus they master the art of cooking. Cooking can be a psychological expression, as food and psychology are interconnected. Another possible psychological explanation why Arabs have mastered the art of cooking is as a response to the oppression in their lives. That can also be seen among other ancient cultures like the Chinese or Indian culture. They have great cooks as well. Perhaps cooking can also be an outlet for the spirit that has been pressured.

People have a natural tendency to express themselves freely. If they do not have such means, they must find a substitute. Food can be a substitute for the expression of bottled up emotion, or it can be an outlet for repressed materials in the unconscious mind. Food also can be an outlet for the expression of psychological difficulty. That can be seen clearly among obese people; food acts as an agent of soothing to their psychological difficulty. Food can serve many purposes. It nurtures the soul, and if not then Arabs seek other means to fulfill the psychological hunger from which most of Arab society suffers.

Putting people down. A cultural practice malfunction among Arabs is putting people down, even among family members. This practice shows the dark side of the Arab soul. Even if the put-down is meant as a joke, the psychological explanation is that it is a survival technique. In other words, I will not allow you to be ahead of me because then you will have whatever you want, and by the time I come along there is nothing left for me. Arabs do not want to see others ahead of them. Undoubtedly, Arab culture is not a positive one, and the dynamic of putting people down is almost embedded in the psyche of the individual. This is not encouraging cultural practices, and that might be a partial reason for Arab's depressive state of being. For example, Gadaffi put down other Arab leaders in almost every Arab convention, and the response was mere laughter. Only King Abdullah of Saudi Arabia was assertive and rejected Gadaffi's insult.

The Law of Retaliation. The law of retaliation has been in the fabric of Arab culture for thousands of years. This part of the desert tradition states if someone kills a member of your family, then you have to take revenge and kill the killer. The rule of the law is not strong enough in desert life; this is why people feel they have to take the law into their own hands. Moreover, Arab culture is still considered a tribal culture. This is the core of that tradition—**settle the conflict by the dagger**. Normally, Arab individuals carry the hate inside of them for many years and they wait for the proper time to take their revenge. A psychological analysis of this shows there was a narcissistic injury at the time of the insult, and perhaps the ego was wounded. Therefore, the individual is unable to tolerate the inner conflict, and has to resort to revenge. Normally, Arab society reinforces that attitude.

Personal compliments. Another cultural practice is personal compliments. Everyone needs compliments, they tend to boost self-esteem, and it may produce a soothing feeling about the world around us. Arabs are ambivalent about this; we want compliments but at the same time we do not accept them easily, because Arabs think complimenting people should be done in their absence not when they are present. However, it does not make sense to compliment people in their absence, because the whole point is that we need the subject of our compliment to hear it, not someone else! Compliments therefore are not well received in Arab culture. Perhaps Arabs are shy about it. However, Arabic literature is filled with compliments to the rulers. Most of those compliments were fantastic and make the rulers even better than a slice of bread, as in reality these rulers were ruthless to the bone. That is part of the hypocrisy in Arab culture. Often, people are naïve enough to believe the compliment and act upon it.

Weaning processes. The process of weaning away from family attachments may take longer for Arabs. They may stay attached to the family for a long time. Females especially, may keep the **umbilical cord connected to their mother**, even if she gets married and has her own children. This practice has been encouraged by the family, and the consequences of this practice can be a deprivation of personal growth. However, this is partially a universal human phenomenon. People do not like to leave their nests. However, an Arab family may encourage the individual to stay in the same house, even if he gets married or has children. Thus, the extended family is necessary in Arab culture because they are inclined to help each other. Normally, family members may put all the resources of the family together so they can pull each other's weight. It can be a very helpful practice in a society with limited resources.

Swaddling. Swaddling children is still a common practice in Arab the world. This involves depriving the child of the use of his limbs, by enveloping them in an endless length of bandage. The skin is sometime excoriated, and the flesh is compressed, almost to the state of gangrene. Circulation is nearly arrested, and the child is without the slightest power of motion. This is convenient to adults so they rarely pay attention to infants. Recent medical studies of swaddling has shown that swaddled infants are extremely passive, their hearts slow down, they cry less, they sleep far more, and in general they are withdrawn and inert. Arabs do this customarily and treat a baby like a parcel for the sake of convenience.

Lying. A sad practice in Arab culture is lying. Arabs lie from morning until evening. Everyone is lying to each other, for the primary reason that without lies, you cannot get what you want. Thus, one must create drama in order to get what he/she needs. It is a part of the fabric of society, as the culture of the Arab is the culture of fears. If a person is fearful inevitably, he will lie. Telling the truth can jeopardize the well being of the individual; for example if a person is engaged in some activities that the rules do not allow, he then has to lie about it. Although it is not healthy practice, I would say a person is forced by society to do so. Otherwise, they would not be able to survive in such an unfair world.

Daily greetings. A silly practice is the daily greeting, in which people greet each other with the body only, with many kisses that do not mean anything. It is a matter of custom; you may even greet people you hate. Analysis of this shows that fear is the primary motive, because Arab society is very closed. People know each other, so you have to save face by being friendly even with those you cannot tolerate.

The other cultural condition relating to greetings is that Arabs are not a happy people in general. They tend to frown; a smile is not part of the cultural practice. You have to be serious in order to be respected; even laughter is not preferred at times. A "sulky face" is an indication of being powerful and serious, so people do not get close to you. For example, rarely do you see a leader of the Arab people with a smile on his face.

Honor. Another cultural practice is that the honor of the family has been placed on the vagina of woman. If she loses her virginity then the whole family is in deep trouble. She may bring shame to the family for the rest of their lives.

However, a paradox exists regarding women in Arab society. On one hand, her sexuality is over valued, while on the other her place in society is less than a male. Moreover, in some Arab countries they may kill the woman if she ever loses her virginity. Although, this practice used to be implemented severely, while now a day people are more relaxed over female virginity, or over the whole concept of honor.

Negativity. Most people know that negative thinking is a protection against possible disappointment. Unfortunately, Arab people view themselves negatively; it is almost as if there is a sense of defeat the majority carries within themselves. If an outsider listens to any casual conversations among Arabs, they may hear a conversation loaded with negative demeaning messages about Arab cultural practices, as well as about themselves. There are many analyses for this. Since Arabs have lived under despot rulers, they have inevitably developed negative views of themselves, because they have been humiliated and disrespected for such a long time. The other analysis for such negative views is that they are surrounded by limited natural resources, because they live in a barren land on the desert, offering them only sand and stones. The last reason for being negative is that Arabs often compare themselves with the rest of the world. They see the world is moving fast and sadly enough they are left behind. All these factors have contributed to make the Arab individual view himself negatively.

Overvaluing the Past. Yet another common cultural practice, Arabs overvalue their heritage and the relics of the past. They focus on the past and if you engage in any conversation, immediately they take you to the past; they have strong nostalgic feelings about it. They do not live in the present. That is understandable, because the past of the Arab was a glorious one and the present is painful and bitter. Thus, they go to the past, writing poetry and books about the past and how the Arabs were powerful and progressive people. Undoubtedly, that was true at the time of the Islamic Renaissance, during which Arabs conquered many countries and built a wonderful prosperous empire. The past may provide them with some psychological comfort and lift their bruised spirits. This fondness for the past means they do not appreciate the present.

Belief in Fate and Destiny. The cultural practice of fate, in which everything is predetermined from the religious perspective as to the truth, has prevalence in Arab society. Nevertheless, individual initiative is strongly needed to make things happen.

Unfortunately, in some instances the Arab individual can submit completely to fate and thus does not have a drive to do things. He may have tried before and reached a dead end, and thus became discouraged. There are many things in the lives of the Arab individual that they cannot do, unless they have a connection or know people in the right place, to help them achieve.

If there are no connections, then it is a struggle to get what are supposedly everyone's rights and privileges. This is why most have a strong belief in fate. They have tried something that did not work, so they say it is fate. Undoubtedly, that can have a soothing effect on painful reality.

All humans have some sort of belief in destiny; Arabs are no exception. However, the Arab may over do it, because of the inability to control the sequence of events in life. Often, lives are controlled by forces beyond individual control, such as by rulers or community leaders, or even by the tyrannical roles of society. As indicated earlier, Arab society is a collectivist society; the roles of the group supersede the desires of the individual. This is why the Arab leaves it to destiny in order to achieve some psychological fulfillment. Otherwise, the inability to control what happens in life can leave an individual seriously disturbed. Arabs hang onto destiny as a defense mechanism to partially alleviate anxiety about what has happened to them.

Envy. Being envious is a universal phenomenon, but it is more pronounced in Arab life. The root cause of this envy is that the majority of Arabs suffer from a shortage of food and other commodities. Arabs are envious over others' camels, or sheep or cows or something else, which they believe should belong to them. This is a mild form of paranoid thinking, or a part of narcissistic tendencies; the Arab wants the whole for himself and no one else can have what he has.

Blame syndrome. The blaming syndrome in Arab culture is closely related to the Arab's inability for self-awareness. If one is aware of his responsibility and his contribution to any action, one accepts that. However, if unaware, one tends to blame others for those contributions. That can be a very easy way to escape responsibility. Arabs by nature are externally oriented people. Hence, if one accepts the responsibility then he has to change the course of action, and that can be a very difficult task to assume. It is very easy to blame someone else for unfortunate circumstances.

Normally, Arabs externalize anything, so the whole society is blaming one another. This behavior is modeled after the head of the family or the head of the community. For example, Arabs have not seen any governmental official admit responsibility for any mistakes. Thus, people believe they have no say over their own actions or behavior.

Even the Arabic language reflects placement of blame. For example if walking and holding a plate and the plate falls and breaks, other languages would say, "I broke the plate". The Arabic language would say the plate is broken, as if the plate did it by itself. That is a funny way to look at it, but that is the reality of the Arabic language.

Pecking order. As long as there has been a societal hierarchy, there have been people who are at the top of the ladder, while others are at the bottom. This "pecking order" is visible in Arab society. Although it probably exists in every society, it is more pronounced in Arab society, due to the absence of societal order to regulate relationships among its members. Moreover, individual appreciation in Arab society is not built on humanistic values; rather it is based on many criteria that calculate the benefit and losses of such transactions.

Hypocrisy. Hypocrisy means that you act the opposite of what you believe. For example, you may not like your neighbor, but you manifest friendly attitudes toward him. Or you do not like the government but you always speak favorably about them. This may come from fear of facing your neighbor, because he may have some power over you or he is well connected, and he may harm you. So, you pretend that you are friendly and loving towards him, to protect yourself.

This cultural practice is seen in almost every aspect of Arab society. Even the word "hypocrisy" is used widely in daily conversation. Once the roles of laws are established, however, and the Arab individual becomes more assertive, there is no place for such behavior in society.

Cajoling others can be a common practice in the Arab world. It is a necessity in order to survive the world of daily transactions.

Being obsequious is also very common. One must ingratiate himself to the people in power and abuse the people considered "below" him. It is obvious at every level of Arab daily life.

Respect for old age. Part of the psychological makeup of an Arab is the respect of elders. Age is equated with acquiring wisdom, and the very existence of gray hair can give the elder individual prestige over others. It is a wonderful and healthy cultural practice in Arab society, while we may see the opposite in the West, where elders are placed in nursing homes. The Arab world is limited in its ability to care for elders outside the family unit. Therefore, the family takes full responsibility of elderly members.

Courage. Arabs are often faced with challenges, and they are up to these challenges. In some instances, Arabs are fearless. This is possibly due to their long history of waging war, so life for them is either to live in dignity or not at all. Historically, Arabs are excellent fighters or warriors. Unfortunately, today despot rulers are trying very hard to "tame" them into a docile people.

Helping family and relatives. One of the highlights of Arab cultural practices is the willingness to help each other—mainly family and relatives. Psychologically, Arabs live with shortages of food, water and other commodities. Thus, when they possess those commodities, they have to share it with the people around them; one day they may need those people, because nothing is stable in their lives.

Islam instructs people to be giving to family and relatives, with the promise of a great reward from God. Therefore, it is not just social solidarity, but a religious obligation that Prophet Mohammad (peace be upon Him) asked of the people. They are to do it for others without expecting any earthly reward; the reward will be from Almighty God. This cultural practice has alleviated a lot of suffering among those who do not have much. In the Arab world, governmental institutions are not established to fulfill the needs of the individual members of society, as they are in the West, so this generosity serves a great purpose.

A sense of belonging. As seen in the previous chapter, Arab society is group-oriented. Thus, a sense of belonging is quite pronounced in the culture. That has some psychological benefit for the individual, as people in every culture like to belong to a group, community, or family at large. A sense of belonging can take away one's loneliness, and may give inner satisfaction that he is a valued member, wanted by his group or community. The sense of belonging functions as a buffer against the alienation that the majority of the human community is feeling in these times.

Chapter Ten

Arab Family Structures

Child Rearing Practices

Your children are not your children.
They are the sons and daughters of life's belonging for itself.
They come through you but not from you.
And though they are with you, yet they belong not to you.
You may give them your love but not your thoughts.
You may house their bodies but not their soul.
You may strive to be like them, but seek not to make them like you.

Kahlil Gibran

The family is the core unit of any society. In the Arab world family plays an extremely important role in building the self-concept of the individual. There are many psychological practices that shape a person and how he/she may play out his life in the real world. For example, if we look to Arab family boundaries, we see it is very rigid. Family members do not allow the individual to interact freely with the outside world, while the relationships among family members are fused. There is no internal boundary; they are overly involved in each other's lives. There is no place for individuality or privacy, and often the family has total say over the affairs of each member. That may be an adaptive response to the family being powerless. If you are powerless you may need to have some control over someone else. And the family members are the closest over which to practice such control.

A positive Oedipus complex can be seen in the Arab family, in that the Son tends to identify with his father, and sometimes there is a disregard for women in the family. That comes from the historical discrimination toward women, wherein women are considered a source of shame. Since the father is the dominant figure in the family that tips the balance in the family and makes the children envoys of his role. He may see the whole family as his property.

The Arab family is **patriarchal**. Because of domination by the father, the upbringing of the child is tyrannical by temperament. However, there have been slight changes lately in the Gulf area of the Arab world, whereby the mother is becoming the center of the family.

The superego may grow stronger in an Arab family, because the overt adherence to the religious practices may put the individual in conflict between his desires, wishes, impulses and the religious practices. That conflict can be seen clearly in the lives of an Arab family.

Arab children are frightened by ghosts or by the dark, or any other scary figures. This can have serious implications for their psychological development. Moreover, Arab families do not respect children and normally do not allow them in the presence of the elders. Unfortunately, children are not treated with dignity or consideration.

Another practice in child rearing is swaddling which is wrapping the baby tightly with lyses bandages. This can result in serious developmental problems for the child who learned, from the early years of life, that he is confined, and his movement is restricted. That may lead to bed wetting, as a child develops some sort of revenge at his family from his early years by urinating over them metaphorically.

There is serious trouble in Arab child rearing, in that most of the time a male child is overly protected by the family—mainly by the mother. She does not allow males to experience any sort of adventure. If he initiates doing something unusual, like climbing a mountain, such risks will be prevented. Since he is surrounded by fears, he grows up cowardly and lacking initiative. Because of constantly hearing "don't do it, you will get hurt", his creativity is stifled and his psychological growth is crippled by fears.

As far as the female child is concerned, the situation is more severe. She is not even allowed to go out of the house in some Arab societies. This is one of the reasons why the Arab world does not have a great female athlete. The females' movements in Arab society are mostly restricted. Some Arab countries do not allow females to play any sort of sport or navigate life alone. Sadly, they see females as weak persons who always need assistance, and protection from the predator, who is the male.

The hierarchy in the Arab family is clearly defined. The head of the family has absolute power over the rest of the family. The head of the tribe can have great influence over many people, because everyone is looking for protection. If you do not have the tribe to protect you, people may take advantage of you. Arab society in general is a tribal one, and often disputes can be settled by the tribal system rather than by the government.

A certain amount of aggression can be seen in the Arab family because an individual's opinion is rarely respected. Thus, family members may be frustrated and angry most of the time. Undoubtedly, the anger among females is more pronounced because she feels clearly that the male in the family is valued more then she. He has more choices than she, as well as having the upper hand over her. Surely, this situation makes her an angry individual.

There is a pecking order in the Arab family. The average father is out hassling with the world to get bread on the table for his family, and he may encounter all sorts of humiliation & abuse. Therefore, when he returns home to his family, he has to find an outlet for his frustrations. Of course he can not find a better or safer place then his home and his family members.

Verbal abuse also exists in the Arab family. Family members may demean each other, perhaps not for malicious reasons, but just for lack of etiquette, lack of awareness or sheer ignorance. In general the Arab family is not a psychologically healthy family.

In Arab society there is an obligation among family members that they should help each other, financially and otherwise. This is actually a great practice. Because the resources of the family are limited in most instances, members must help each other. This family dynamic can have advantages and disadvantages to individual members. It may help the family in serious need, or it may drown the individual in concern if he is unable to pull himself from such burdensome obligations for life.

Overall, the Arab family does not encourage autonomy; instead they encourage dependency and control. To maintain cohesiveness, all family members must demonstrate compliance, due to the lack of education among most of the family. On the other hand, this can be a great psychological support to family members. As we indicated early in other chapters, Arab society is a collectivist one. The focus is rather on the whole community, not on the individual.

Trust can be an issue in Arab society. Children are taught mistrust of others, and to not put confidence in anyone. They are told, "Just hold your cards tight to your chest".

Another issue regarding the Arab family is the practice of saving face or the good name of the family. Members must never do anything that may bring the shame to the reputation of family. Thus, an individual may live in constant conflict just to do what the family wants him to do, and to not veer from the norms of the family. Often such behavior takes away the essence of the individual.

A wonderful practice in the Arab family is great respect to the elderly family members. We often see just the opposite in the West. Older persons with gray hairs have some influence in the community and over young people. Normally, Arabs revere old age, as they see it as bringing wisdom and better judgment.

The other helpful practice among Arab families is to have social solidarity. They help each other financially and they stand by any member who is in need. They are similar to the Italian family in America when they immigrated in last century. The bank did not loan them money, so they stood by each other and they leaned on each other to start their businesses.

Another example of social solidarity is in Moroccan families. They often adopt needy children, even though they themselves are in serious financial needs. Somehow they manage to make it work. Moroccan families will also cook couscous on Fridays and take it to the local Mosques to feed poor people. These are great practices, cherished in Arab society.

The weaning process in the Arab family takes longer than usual. Thus an individual may stay un-weaned from the family group all his life. They are entangled perpetually in the family organization. Therefore, we see fewer people who are independent of the family. Undoubtedly, this contributes to the neuroses of individuals.

Obviously, there are a great number of Arabs who are not fully developed emotionally, because of their neurotic attachment to their family. It is also counterproductive to the whole society, because the individual has no time left for developing a friendship with other people or "discovering" himself/herself. The center of life is the family. This why we see great numbers of Arab individuals think "inside the box", not from the outside, because the family has encouraged prolonging the infantile stage of intellectual/emotional development.

In summary, Freud has encapsulated the whole concept of rearing a child in one statement **[child who has bountiful mother's love can stand all the vicissitudes of life]**. Thus, mother is the cornerstone of all aspects of a child's development.

Chapter Eleven

The Psychology of Emotion

Emotional Expression

All human beings have reservoirs of emotions, and as we grow in life, we go through many stages of cultivation and negotiation to channel our emotion into proper perspectives. The emotional aspect in Arab culture inclines toward the extremes of expression; either calm and relaxed, or angry and hostile, with often nothing in between. If you observe an argument among Arabs, it might appear they may kill each other right away, but the Arab language is loaded with empty rhetoric. Eventually they kiss each other and leave.

There are myriad examples regarding the extreme expression of emotion in the daily lives of Arab people. Arabs may express overwhelming love, and at the same time express profound hate or vengeance. This may puzzle outside observers. It is the result of bottled up emotions and pent up anger, due to living in an oppressive society. Arabs have not learned to negotiate their emotions within their lives. Emotional expression is a very fine skill, which needs to be learned either at home or at school. In the

Arab world normally, neither homes nor schools are equipped to teach people emotional management skills.

Emotional expression in the Arab culture is very much intertwined with the entire psychological structure of the individual. For example, non-educated people may display Alexithymic traits (the lack of expression). Educated people vent their emotions verbally.

Arabs may exhibit anger and hostility because of abuse from society, family, and mostly governmental institutions. Thus, they tend to "jump" at you if you become involved in any discussion, and they get "heated up" easily.

If we examine the emotional part of Arab culture, there is a certain amount of emotional immaturity, because Arabs are centered on themselves. If there is any perceived slight that may touch their vulnerability, they erupt like a volcano and then you see the stream of emotion pouring out. Normally, people can develop emotional maturity when they train and go through many trials in emotional expressions. Then they may reach a certain amount of maturity.

Arab emotions are crude and may require some refinement, but perhaps that has a positive side to it. For example, if an Arab woman loves someone, she may give all her heart to the lover. She has not had an emotional outlet, and once she finds one she may give herself totally.

Look how Arab society socializes men and women differently in their emotional expression. Females are encouraged to express emotions that elicit support and reflect weakness, such as fear, unhappiness, and helplessness. Men, on other hand, are encouraged to express emotions that encourage action, such as anger, anxiety and revenge. Thus, the Arab woman may suffer in silence just to keep the coherence of the family (Abu-Baker, Israel Journal of Psychiatry, 2005).

Family and society do not allow the Arab individual to develop his own emotional maturity. The family often thinks for the individual, or provides a ready answer for concerns or problems. The Arab individual often has a stream of emotion, and he does not know how to channel it properly.

Arabs are very courageous people; they have been trained for thousands of years to fight in wars, from the small tribal war to a local fight with the neighbors. It is easy to arouse their emotion and pump them up for any action. In this can be seen a certain degree of impulsiveness, too.

One of the other salient emotional characteristics of the Arab is the ability to carry hatred for many years. They have been trained for vengeance since the early years in their lives by family and society.

Arabs in general are inclined to rush to judgment without listening or gathering the facts. The emotional part of the self surfaces right away and takes over the logical part of the self. Since the whole culture is a verbal culture, listening is not part of it. The individual is encouraged to answer right away, or otherwise lose the verbal battle. It is common to see several people talking at the same time with no one listening. Each individual is thinking ahead to what the answer might be, or each is busy in his own private mental dialogue.

The Arab people in general are depressed and anxious, because they lack security and face uncertainty in their daily lives. Thus, they can be harsh in their expression and sometimes even abusive verbally or physically to each other. The sad reality of Arab culture is they have not lived stable, secure lives throughout history. That has very serious and lethal ramifications in their personality makeup. The mistrust in their surroundings and themselves is very clear, and consequently they are very frustrated, confused and have chronic anger.

If you initiate a casual conversation with an Arab, he will immediately engage you in an endless complaint about many things. They draw a very negative picture about their reality and the lives of others. In this regard, other nationalities need to be compassionate, not blame them for their negativity. Their lives have been a constant struggle for survival and to ensure basic daily needs, let alone security or stability.

Psychologically speaking if you see injustices all your life and cannot change them, you become angry, frustrated and disappointed at your own world as well as the world around you.

The Arab individual is naïve in his emotional expression and if you give him compliments, he will give you the shirt off his back. His personality is influenced by many factors like society, religion, government, social order and family structures. Thus, he feels that he is torn apart by all theses factions, as well as between the traditional and modern life.

Arabs like to possess power because they have been living powerless lives for thousands of years. Collectively and individually, power has been assigned to family, the elite class of society, political systems and tribal hierarchy.

When you walk down a street in the Arab world, you observe that people frown or sulk. They are depressed; even the news broadcaster on TV has this expression. Smiling is not part of the Arabs' emotional expression. Arabs are unhappy people because of their painful circumstances, which have greatly influenced them. Consequently, many have a callous heart.

The world has witnessed a lot of torture of political prisoners in the Arab world. Historically, it is said that the Arabs invented the techniques of torture. Today's rulers such as Saddam, Gadaffi, Assad, and Ali Saleh of Yemen, Bin Ali of Tunisia or Mubarak of Egypt are some of the most ruthless rulers in the history of mankind. They have inflicted unimaginable pain and suffering on their people, and that pain will last for many generations.

If you examine Arabic literature, you find that much has been written about pain and suffering. There is a plethora of novels regarding disappointment and pain. Therefore, it is highly probable that an Arab will possess an existential philosophy view that life is a painful journey, and one must learn to cope with it.

Arabs are judgmental; they volunteer to give advice and criticism, with a complete disregard for an individual's beliefs or opinions. They assume guardianship over people, much like the privileges of being the father for everyone, without any permission from others. That gives the individual who engages in such practice some Ego satisfaction, and perhaps may give him an edge over other people.

Trapped or oppressed people frequently become deceptive and manipulative, or slavish and dependent, or all of these things, in order to keep from getting hurt more. Arabs have considered themselves trapped for a long time; this is why part of their behavior is manipulative.

In conclusion, the prerequisite for people to become truly visible to one another, to trust one another, to grow to love one another, and to have healthy attitudes, is to feel safe within his heart. Psychological liberty must be assured, for this is the backbone for any social and political emancipation.

Chapter Twelve

Psychological Structure of Arab Society

The Characteristics of the Arab People

Are there any specific characteristics for Arabs, or Brazilians, or Cubans? Absolutely. There are certain cultural practices, which can shape both the conscious and subconscious of people without them even being aware of such influence. These cultural practices can seep into the psyche of people and become a "remote control", moving them around accordingly. Individuals interact daily with their surroundings and mutual influence can take place within the deep recesses of the personality.

Here are a few of the characteristics of the Arab people. Arab society is collectivist; the individual derives his self-concept from the group, family or community to which he belongs. His personal success, failure and accomplishments stem from the way society views him. He has to belong to either a large or a small group, either a tribe or an immediate family, and that may define his place in society. For example, if one is born to an influential or wealthy family, he can sail through life with less difficulty. If one is born to a less fortunate family he may face many obstacles and difficulties in life, and has to work very hard to overcome the hurdles which exist. The fortunate person from an influential family may apply less energy in order to have what they desire.

Arab society is a shame-based culture. This is unique to Arab culture, and an individual must be mindful not to do anything that may bring shame upon the family or the community. This can be more pronounced with females; a woman should protect her sexuality, and not lose her virginity until married. Most of the time shame is associated with sexuality. Arabs are obsessed with female sexuality, and may have paranoid ideas regarding it. Consequently, there are many restrictions on women's daily habits and movements. The hidden message regarding women is, please just keep them under control; otherwise, they may bring shame to their families.

An outside observer may see such beliefs as archaic and useless for life in the 21st century. However, this cultural practice has lasted for thousands of years, and cannot go away or be erased from people's conscious mind that easily.

Arab culture is also guilt-ridden, because of their adherence to ritualistic behavior established over thousands of years. In turn, that breeds some neurotic tendency of guilt within the individual, i.e., the individual may do something that is diametrically opposed to what he believes. Constant struggles and conflict within the individual push the guilt to the surface. Often, the family uses this guilt to manipulate and control individual members.

The Arab suffers from a serious case of Ego arrested development, because of rigid roles and practices. Thus, the individual may stay in the infantile stage of development, which means he is hungry for validation and approval by others. That can have detrimental effects on an individual's ability to be a healthy, capable member of society. Hence, society does not encourage a person to actualize his own potential. In fact, Arab society may stifle individual initiative and keep people stagnant. Therefore, collectively the Arab people lack personal initiative or creativity. Unfortunately, Arabs are thus described as a backward people in their personal development, and their contributions to the human community are minimal. Educated Arabs loudly harangue that change in the structure of society must take place, so society can move forward and Arabs can become active participants in global development. Thus far, their cries are to no avail, because there are forces in society that prefer to keep people in total darkness and isolation. These forces—the elite class and the rulers—thrive in the midst of such ignorance.

Arabs are also inclined to be self-absorbed, because they are not critical or reflective of themselves. That is due to the orientation of Arab society, which is outward, not inward. In the outward society, the individual is always trained to focus on pleasing others, or on superficial appearances. As a result, the individual loses his personality and becomes an echo or reflection of others. It is a paradox, because the individual must focus outside himself, but on the other hand, he may feel neglected regarding his own personal needs, and thus turns inward and becomes self-absorbed.

Arab society is blame-based. Any wrongdoing is attributed to outside forces, and personal responsibility is never taken for any action. This is a counterproductive defense mechanism and certainly leads to poor insight. Since Arabs are externally oriented, blaming others is part of the structure of society. Such attitudes do not allow the individual to look inside himself and accept responsibility for his own actions.

Sadly, blaming others for failure or inability deprives people of the unique opportunity to accept challenges and move forward. A ludicrous example illustrates how blame is imbedded in daily lives. During a television interview, the Agriculture Minster of Iraq was asked why there are no eggs in the markets. His answer was that the chickens stopped producing eggs; he was unable to accept the shortages in the market as being a result of his poor management. He blamed it on the chickens!

Arabs tend to hold onto the past, because the past was glorious, mainly during the Islamic Renaissance. Thus, there is an absence of modern institutions. Arabs may harbor bitterness today because of disappointment, colonization, despot leaders and a lack of technological advancement. There are poems written about the past and how the Arab conquered the whole world; that was a golden age to them. Perhaps there is a certain amount of fixation on the past to assuage today's anxiety about the future and the yearning for liberation.

Another element to Arab society's structure is that everyone must accept duties and responsibilities without question. That has bred many neuroses within Arab society. An individual in the Arab culture is merely a person who fulfills without questioning, the duties that society dictates. Complaints regarding cultural practices are a prerequisite to being accepted and approved by society. It can be a very subtle dynamic with some psychological fulfillment for the individual, through a sense of belonging. However, it may be a shallow fulfillment.

The Arab people in general are not trusting; probably due to false promises they have heard for many years from their fathers, authority figures or community leaders. Doubt is therefore part of the society's structure; everyone is lying to everyone else, and the truth has been lost in the process.

A salient feature of Arab psychology is fear; Arabs have a fear-based culture. The populace is fearful of metaphoric castration by rulers. If a person is frightened, he will try to fight back to quiet his own fears. This creates a vicious cycle in that an individual is fearful and in order to quiet that fear, he must lash out or project his fears onto others.

The other essential fear in the Arab personality is the fear of judgment by others; **Kalam Alnass** is the Arabic word for it. Arab culture is a judgmental culture and anything a person does is subject to judgment. That can induce many fears inside the individual. Hence, such judgment can have serious consequences on individual lives. Avoiding such judgment can be the constant preoccupation of people, almost as if the entire culture is paralyzed by Kalam Alnass. In other words, all of the people in Arab society are hostages of each other.

Overall, Arabs are burdened by the heavy weight of their cultural practices, many of which have a complete disregard for personal wishes, desires or respect for individuality. Thus, the average Arab is frustrated, anxious and depressed, and maintains a tone of anger at himself and at the establishment.

The Arab interpretation of respect is another troubling character in the Arab personality. Normally people are respected according to a specific criteria or their place in society. If they are from an influential or wealthy family, have political affiliations, or have some connections with people in power, they are respected. Arabs do not respect individuals merely because they are human; they have to have some status and influence in society. Otherwise, they are treated as insignificant and marginal people who happen to be living there.

The notion of people as masters of their own destiny is still alien to the Arab people; individuality and uniqueness are strange concepts. Arab society prefers the roles of community over individual desires. Undoubtedly, that causes the individual to be in constant conflict with society, as well as with himself.

Average Arabs are gullible. One of most salient characteristics of this aspect of personality is excessive admiration of others, and dependency on them. Arab culture has created the cult of personality and most Arabs have an idol in their lives. Arabs almost worship people, such as community figures and others who have influence over their lives. The Arab family encourages dependency and prolongs the infantile stage of development; consequently, the individual may become naïve, with immature judgment. Another part of being gullible is to easily accept any thoughts or ideas presented, without questioning the validity of such thoughts or ideas. Questioning the unwritten roles of a tyrannical society may have an effect on the cohesiveness of that society. Eventually, society may consider the questioner a heretic or iconoclast, and the questioner's life may be in jeopardy

The Arab individual lives in constant conflict and contradiction. The conflict concerns wishes, desires and hope, which reality does not fulfill. Thus, an individual stays in a stage of psychological deprivation, which can have serious psychological ramifications on both the individual and society. Contradictions occur because the individual has two systems of values: the private one that allow the individual to do what his heart may tell him to do, and the societal, buying into what society sells him. Often those systems come into clash with one another.

A person is unable to tolerate such internal contradictions, and thus people may become extremely angry for a minor slight.

For example, in his private system a person can do anything that is opposed to the principle of religion. In the societal system, he appears to show people that he is a virtuous human being. A person may live all his life in such contradiction and conflict, with the result that Arabs are self-centered, envious and rather rude to each other.

These conflicts and contradictions have contributed to the emergence of an unhealthy and confused personality—a dual or split personality. An Arab can hold two different sets of values that can completely oppose each other, at the same time. For example, a person may preach all day long about religion and the value of adherence to the ethics and teachings of religion. However, at night he may go drink alcohol and do other things that contradict these religious values. Interestingly enough, he never sees anything wrong with such contradictions, and assumes there is a clear separation between the two sets of values. Privately, that makes the individual unhappy because he may see there is no alignment between the act and the beliefs.

This type of personality split is similar to the Dr.Jekyll/ Mr. Hyde personalities well known in Western literature. He is the same person but acts completely different in different circumstances; that is what has transpired in the Arab personality. Arabs' perception of wrong and right is flummoxed by their belief system. The personality has split and seems to be operating on two different tracks, the first being old-fashioned morals, the other corrupt and deceitful behavior.

There is a certain amount of dogma about many things in the Arabs' belief system, and there is no flexibility. They view their lives with a great deal of rigidity. Often, the system of logic does not operate, because emotionality overcomes their logic. Thus, we see a lot of poor judgment in people's daily transactions. Many people will rush to offer advice and try to show others as fools, and contend they have better judgment. This very unhealthy dynamic takes place often in Arabs' daily lives.

Since Arab society is collectivist, Arabs tend to think only "within the box". Group thinking is more valued than individual thinking. In general, Arabs are like parrots; they repeat what others say without questioning the validity of those thoughts. Thinking within the box is archaic, and can be outdated. Humanity's progress has not been through this type of thinking. Most of the people responsible for the progress and development of the human race are those who have gotten out of the box and frequently shattered it to pieces. Undoubtedly, Arabs need a serious case of self-reflection, and reassessment of their whole value system in terms of relating to each other, and relating to the world around them. Perhaps, this book will shed some light on the dysfunction that has plagued Arab society for a long time.

Chapter Thirteen

The Dynamic of Oppression

Higher Self & Lower Self

Human individuals are not born a blank slate as many behavior scientists profess. We are born with a certain potential for being benevolent or mischievous; good or evil, [we have both sides; Mother Teresa & Saddam]. And, that may depend upon two factors—the environment into which we were born, like our parental upbringing as well as the genetic predisposition. If the environment is healthy and our parents are aware of their crucial roles, then our contributions to ourselves as well as to our fellow humans can be uplifting and promoting. If the environment is impoverished in many aspects and our parents are ignorant, then we grow up with serious psychological limitations. As far as genetic inclination, perhaps the intervention here is limited.

We can be more specific about the meaning of those two aspects of our personality. The good, or the benevolent, part we might call "the higher self," and the mischievous part we might call "the lower self." Moreover, these concepts were clearly stated in all the books of religions. Thus, there is always a struggle inside every individual between the higher self and the lower self.

The higher self can be defined as the disposition or the inclination to the sense of justice, forgiveness, freedom, caring about others, compassion, helpfulness, being giving, and respect for fellow humans. On the other hand, the lower self is characterized by the tendency of being envious, jealous, aggressive, selfish, violent, greedy, lazy, and oppressive of others.

This question may present itself: How do we communicate with sides of the self, the higher and the lower? We may say that it depends upon society, and our parents. For example, if society promotes individual freedom, a sense of justice, kindness, and a respect for law, then we may cultivate this corner of the higher self. And if our parents attend to our emotional needs and value us as human beings, then we grow as healthy individuals. But if society lacks freedom and a sense of justice and parents abuse us then we may tap into the rubbish of the lower self. Hence, the focus of this journey on societal and environment contributions. Because being good parents tends to depend on the individual family in any culture.

Let us examine the application of these two concepts in reality. In the western world, individual freedom exists, the rules of the law are respected and individual rights and privileges are guaranteed. In such cases, the tendency is towards cultivation of the higher self. Consequently, there is a place for creative activities, and members of the society can thrive and flourish. On the contrary, in the Arab world, lack of freedom and a sense of justice may bring the characteristics of the lower self out in full swing, showing in jealousy, envy, aggression, lack of respect for human values, and a lack of creativity.

There is one caveat that needs to be made. The presentation is not an absolute sense regarding western or eastern societal characteristics; it is just in relative terms. No doubt, the western society has its own deficits, and it can tap into the lower self at times. And, the Arab society may tap into the higher self at times. But, the overall observations are that the western society has evolved to address the needs of the higher self, while the Arab society is still not ambitious enough to tackle those needs.

Fundamentally speaking, if a society lacks freedom, which is considered the antidote for the human soul, individuals will show the repulsive side of their personality. The lack of freedom and the oppression in the Arab world has brought the worst out of the people. This is why we see the dark side of the Arab individual prevailing these days.

Constitutionally, Arabs are not a bad people, but oppression throughout their long history has marginalized their personalities and has twisted their perceptions. Thus, they became the source of disturbance to themselves as well as to others.

The kernel of truth is that each individual inherently carries the seed of corruption as well as the seed of goodness in his / her personality makeup. Which seed grows depends upon the ground on which the seed falls. Because of the oppression and lack of freedom, the Arab society has fertile ground in which the seed of corruption can germinate and has been the norm of their lives. It has stripped the Arab individual of his humanity and left him empty with eyes wide open for revenge and aggression. This is why freedom can be the ultimate goal for psychological health and is the panacea for human growth. Freedom is the healer for a lot of societal illness. Freedom and a sense of social justice can bring out the beauty of an individual. This is why we see a lot of intellectual development in the West and its absence in the East. The oppression, the unfair treatment, and the lack of freedom in the Arab world causes the Arab individual to be in a constant of fighting with his family, in the work place, on the street, and within him/herself simply because his needs, desires, and wishes have not been fulfilled.

Freedom and a sense of justice and equality are not luxuries; they are necessities and indispensable parts of an individual's psychological fulfillments. Western thinkers have recognized that fact for a long time, and they have established and built up a society that nurtures such functions. Arab thinkers, as well, have realized that and sacrificed their lives, but to no avail. Somehow, the oppression became a fabric of Arab society. The challenge for all of people is to weed it out, even though it can be a very colossal task. However, most of the people in Arab society are tired of looking for pieces of bread for their families in spite of the enormous amount of wealth in this part of the world.

As a result of the long history of oppression and lack of freedom in the Arab world, a painful fact presents itself—the Arab psychology became very allergic to freedom and a sense of justice. Even the educated people reject it and say, "Freedom does not fit our society. We are a people always needing to be controlled by iron fist." It's as if the people in this part of the world are wild animals and need to be caged. When people live for such a long time under oppression and the lack of freedom, their minds become fossilized, and they reject anything that may bring them a challenge for growth or development. Because the channel of communication has been directed towards the lower self for a long time, there has been complete negligence of the higher self.

Anyone who works in behavior science understands that there are no bad people or good people. People can have both inclinations, but society may orient its members one way or the other and promote or demote their values. The Arab has been subjected to such treatment for so long that often they do not even question their status quo. They got used to it, and they do not know of or have ever experienced anything different. Although, a large number of them have visited the West, have seen the life there, perhaps, may wish to live that kind of life, but they would not do anything to change their own life. Instead, they merely accept their meaningless existence. The Arab individual has lost his sense of courage; he/she has become psychologically weak and ingratiated their way to the people in power. Painfully, they accepted for themselves to be only voracious consumers of Western materialisms and have not accepted the core values of the West.

The Arab society has been infected by a sense of helplessness because the characteristics of the lower self have been in full operation for such a long time, while the higher self has been dwarfed. In some societies we may sometimes observe struggles between the higher self and the lower self. However, in Arab society, such struggles are very rare. In fact, we may see the complete submission and acceptance of an individual's humiliation.

Conclusions

Each person inherently carries healthy values and pathological values. We may call these the higher self and lower self, or the dark side of the self [the mean self], and the bright side of the self. Our beloved father, Sigmund Freud, called them the superego and the Id. If the surrounding society and parents are healthy, the communication can be directed toward the higher self. That can bring out the best in a person. If the surroundings are unhealthy, the communication tends to take place with the lower self, and that can bring out the worst in a person.

The over-arching wisdom is that a society should structure itself in such a way as to tap into the core of the individual higher self, rather than flirt with the dark side of the soul. At the present time, the Arab society may need a serious self-reflection or self-examination to eradicate the tyranny of the culture and establish a free society. Once a society does that, the higher self will thrive, and the resulting contributions can be immense to the individual as well as to the common good of people.

Chapter Fourteen

East is East . . . West is West, The Twain Shall Never Meet

Alexander Pope English Poet

Often, there are strong arguments prevailing on many levels of society's thinking between the Arab cultures and Western cultures. The core of the arguments is: *What is the difference between both cultures?* Arabs may think of themselves as backward people, or that they are behind the progress of the human community. Or, they may think of themselves as the descendents of the great civilization and have cavalier attitudes.

These arguments are much more pronounced among Arabs than the people of the West. I have lived in both cultures, but I hear it more often in the Arab culture. I would like to give my perspectives as a person who lives in both cultures and as a psychologist who specializes in the interpretation of human behaviors. However, I will try to shed some light on the nature of the differences of the two cultures. Even though the purpose of these arguments is to develop some psychological understanding and appreciation of both cultures, we are aware that there is a chasm between them.

The First Argument

Human beings are born with serious deficits whether in the East or in the West. For example, we are selfish, greedy, and aggressive by nature. God has sent many prophets to cultivate our nature. Some of us are cultivated beings and evolved spiritually, but the majority of us are still unable to transcend beyond our selfish mediocre nature.

In the West they have realized this fact about human nature, and they put in place a lot of laws to manage or control human greed; in the Arab world, however, we are left to our own desires or wishes or whims to be in control of ourselves. We see a lot of poverty in the Arab world even though we have a sufficient wealth. Perhaps, we do not have specific laws to regulate the human selfish tendency. For example, America has the highest number of legislators and institutions in the world to manage human behaviors. If we leave the human being to his own desire or wish, then he will eat alive the people around him, so to speak. It does not seem a romantic view of human nature, but that is the reality. People in the Arab world have an untamed ego; they like to have what their hands may hold. The Western society does not allow an individual person to wander around, letting his unbridled self take over the lot of his fellow human.

Our holy book, the Quran, spells out an insightful story about our human selfish nature. There were two brothers—one had ninety nine goats, and the other one had just one goat. The one with 99 wanted to have the one from his brother so he could have 100 goats, instead of 99. It is a clear indication of our innate human greed. The Western society trains people to follow the rules of law in order to control self-centered tendencies, while the Arab individual has not matured enough to go beyond oneself. Or perhaps, we do not have a specific mechanism to manage our greed. Thus, we are a massively self-absorbed people.

The Second Argument

The Arab culture is a fear-based culture. There are a lot of things that can initiate our fears. In the early years of our life, parents tend to insert tremendous fears of many things into us. For example, my mother used to put me to sleep and, if I did not want to go to sleep, she frightened me with the dark, with Jen, or even with fish; thus, I grew up afraid of the dark and of the fish. When a human being is raised up with such fears, do not expect him/her to be creative. Thus, we are behind the West in science and many fields of knowledge. Basically, we are fearful people. Our soul has been squashed by crippling fears, **mostly the fears of others**. Fears can also bring depression and make us unhappy and gloomy. If any individual operates out of fears, it can bring about all sorts of psychological problems. Perhaps they are not aware of the damage that they inflict upon their children when a family, a society, and a school all conspire to instill fears deep in our conscious or unconscious self.

However, Western society instills courage and hope in their children. The family or the educational system tries to produce a fearless person. Thus, Western individuals tend to experience a lot of adventures in their life. For example, they climb mountains and do all sorts of crazy things which make them very fascinating people. Consequently, the Western person can be creative and forward-thinking, while the Arab individual feels limited and confined by a lot of forces beyond his control. That is a marked difference between the two cultures.

As they say in the field of human motivation, a fearful person loses his role as an effective individual in life. If any individual feels he/she does not have control over his/her life, it can be very detrimental to his/her well-being. Arab people may also suffer from serious boredom, and sometimes they may experience a meaningless existence. If you visit any Arab country and talk with the people, you will reach this sad conclusion.

The Third Argument

The Arab culture does not have an appreciation of the unique, special, or productive individual. It will try to assassinate him/ her psychologically, or try to plot against him, or even to remove him from his place. A creative person might come up with new ideas, and that could be very threatening to the majority because it may show the inadequacy of the rest of us. Because such an individual may constitute a danger, and we have to get rid of him or her, a productive, creative, and sincere person may suffer in the Arab world. Thus, the majority of the scholars in the Arab world seek to live somewhere else and immigrate mainly to the West. They choose to live in the West because the West nurtures their creativity and uniqueness.

Moreover, in the Arab world a hard-working person with good intentions to make a difference may be humiliated and thrown out in disposal. When you speak with people, you will hear a lot of stories supporting this argument. In other words, the Arab culture **tends to bring people down**. On the contrary, the Western culture **tends to bring people up**. For many years I have worked in the West and have experienced this. If a person is unique and serious about making a difference, he tends to be promoted, highly appreciated, and rewarded for his dedication. Western society also tends to focus on productivity and enjoyment. They appreciate anyone who contributes to their development and good life. They use many ways to show you and acknowledge that you are a worthwhile being.

The Fourth Argument

The Arab society is a collectivist society, and the Western society is an individualistic society. What this means in a broad sense is that an individual in a collectivist society tends to drive his self-concept or self-esteem from his community, tribe, organization, and family at large. The individual cannot stand alone. His surroundings are more important then his personality. In other words, an individual in a collectivist society tends to build up the sense of self through the way he is seen in the community or through his place in society. However, in an individualistic society, of which most of the Western world is comprised, an individual tends to develop his sense of self through personal merit and achievement. In the end, regardless of the place of the family, an individual's self-concept is based upon his/her own hard work and accomplishments. Personal identity in the Arab world stems from many factors outside the individual self, while in the West, the identity is shaped by an individual's performance. This is a sharp difference between the two cultures.

We would all like to have a sense of belonging, but it is more pronounced in the Arab than in the Western culture. The individual in the Arab society tries to work hard to please others so he/she can have society's approval. There are also established codes of conduct that individuals must never cross. At birth, the child finds the script already written that he/she must follow. Any violation of the codes can have serious consequences. But in the West, the individual is the one who designs his own code of conduct. This can be confusing at times, but it can also facilitate the creative part of the person. In the West an individual struggles to gain personal recognition, while in the Arab culture, he may inherit or merely be given recognition by his family.

The Fifth Argument

Perhaps related to the Fourth Argument (self-concept in an individualistic v. collectivist society) is that of individual appraisal. An individual in the Arab world tends to be appraised, or evaluated, or respected according to a set of unwritten roles. For example, having an influential family, wealth, and power, are factors that play a part in individual assessment. If a person has more wealth, or more power, or has an influential family, then he/she is respected accordingly. In the West, however, an individual's appraisal is based on personal accomplishment or on individual success.

Perhaps if we are critical in our view, we can see that there is a human element in the way the West looks at the individual because the assessment is based on who you are and what you have done as a human being. In the Arab culture, poor people with no strong family background and no power have limited opportunity. And, such an assessment can strip away an individual's humanity and dignity.

*   *   *

There is an ocean of difference between the two cultures. One culture promotes the skilled person and nurtures his creative self, while the other hinders an individual's spontaneity and stifles his soul.

The five arguments can characterize the prevailing aspects of the two cultures. However, I would like to make clear that no one culture is better than another. But, there are some features that differentiate one from the other. We just need to understand and be mindful of such differences. We must also try to identify the sets of limitations that arise with any culture's practices and see if such practices foster human creativity or deaden the soul. We must never make excuses for or apologize for certain cultural practices that might not facilitate human growth and dignity. We also have to acknowledge that the Arabs contributed greatly to the human community in many fields of science during the Islamic Renaissance. But since then, Arabs have lost the spirit of creativity and the art of giving. Perhaps, the only hope that we have lies in sincere self-reflection and reassessment to our strong hold on dogmatic beliefs about many things in our life. We also need to set our souls free.

There is a final observation that there is some certain hostility from the Arab towards the west, and perhaps, that may result from being envious of the west for what they have, or for their great advancements.

On the other hand we may see a lot people are interested to move to the west, it is dichotomy, there is a love-hate relationship.

And that may depend on the circumstances of the Arab that they go through it.

People in the west have free spirit, thus, they have invented all the modern technology, while people in Arab world are suffocated by many layers of oppressions; the rulers, the tyrannical society, tribal system as well as the rigid roles of the old cultural practices.

Chapter Fifteen

Arab Self image and Identity Formation

The supreme law of life is this: the sense of worth of the self shall not be allowed to be diminished.

Alfred Adler 1946

The Arab self-image and identity can be a mixture of history, religions, cultural practices and family domination. Arabs may develop a false self-image because the individual may see himself as a reflection of his family. Thus he becomes invisible and creates a false sense of self, in an attempt to feel real in his overwhelming world, pulling him in different directions without mercy.

Often the Arab self-image may be associated with the inheritance of a great civilization, as the Arabs regard themselves. Their geographical location has contributed to the feeling of importance.

The Arabs are receivers of their beliefs and experiences, handed down to them from authority figures such as the head of the tribe, the head of the family and the head of the government. Thus, they have secondhand identity, because there is no originality in their contributions of what has been handed down to them.

Often, Arabs are not sure about themselves, and thus tend to repeat themselves to make themselves clear, or to compensate for the confusion within their identity.

There are serious conflicts/contradictions within an Arab individual between the ego ideal and the real self. He may express himself in the loftiest moral tone, but, under proper circumstances, he may also freely descend to a low stratum of moral behavior. As such, Arabs may have dual identity or even triple identity.

As far as the Arab identity crisis, they may feel powerless and are thus inclined to do two things. First, they try to please those on whom they are dependent; second, they attempt to be as much like those in power as possible. Sadly enough, the more they idealize people in power, the more they hate themselves, because in such cases they have lost the essence of their identity. Undoubtedly, that has created identity confusion.

Unfortunately, self-contempt is embedded in the Arab psychology, thus the individual tends to read insult into the most innocent remark. He may respond to his projected self-contempt or frustration within himself by unleashing an acid tongue, or sometimes he may turn his anger back upon himself in the form of chronic anxiety and depression. If you walk down any street in any Arab country, you will see people walking with frowns, because of the sad conditions under which they have been living for such long time.

Furthermore, Arab people may also suffer from a lost identity in the midst of the demands from family, society, and community. Thus, they have many complaints about their lot in life. Individuals are tormented between their desires / wishes and the approval and acceptance of society.

The Arab individual may derive his identity through the sense of belonging to the community. Undoubtedly, such affiliation has its own psychological cost, in that the person must give up some of his personal freedom or creativity to be accommodated by society. Otherwise, he may be outcast or ostracized. That in itself may bring great inner conflict and suffering.

Most Arabs have a serious case of self-absorption, because the surrounding world pushes them to be that way. It is a "dog-eat-dog" world and each must watch out for himself. On the other hand, this is a collectivist society which wants you to adhere to the agreed upon roles and regulations, written or unwritten. Thus, people often are bored with themselves, because there is no self-actualization.

Self-criticism does not exist in Arab culture. All criticism is externalized, i.e., all bad fortune is attributed to an outside force, which is beyond their control. Arabs do not want to assume the responsibility for their own action. This is the main orientation of society. In most instances there are certain forces operating outside the control of the individual. Consequently, the individual may develop a helpless identity or form pathetic attitudes, as his message to himself is, "What is the point? I am uncounted as an active, valuable member of society." Here, we can see a clear crisis of identity within the Arab individual.

The other factor, which has largely contributed to the deformity of the Arab identity, is the domination of authority in every level of life. Since people always must look to authority figures, that does not give them the chance to look to themselves. Thus, they may suffer from a shallow identity, or immaturity. Their value system can be severely twisted. Because of this, they naturally identify with the hostile forces in their society. Thus, this represents an accurate psychological picture of the identity crisis that has prevailed in the Arab world for centuries, and still is today.

Chapter Sixteen

The Psychology of Language

You talk when you cease to be at peace with your thoughts.
And when you can no longer dwell in the solitude of your
heart you live in your lips and sound is a diversion and
pastime.
And in much of your talking, thinking is half murdered.
When you meet your friend on the roadside or in marketplace,
let the spirit in you move your lips and direct your tongue.

—Kahlil Gibran

There is a great association between language and the psychology of culture. Language tends to empower the speaker; he develops a sense of belonging to the large society. Language is the container of our thoughts and can shape cultural identity. Arab culture revolves around the Arabic language; it is embedded into the individual identity. Moreover, the holy book Quran adds to the strength of the Arabic language. Consequently, Arabs feel proud in Islam's requirement that every Muslim around the world must learn Arabic.

However, words just for the sake of words can cause intellectual regression. That has happened in some instances with the Arabic language. There is a type of emotionality in the use of Arabic. When an individual recites poetry or chants, he almost goes into a hypnotic state, thereby affecting the mood and reducing the ability to think clearly.

Often, in Arab gatherings there is debate. That may spiral into rising emotion and sometimes may contribute to discord. However, it is part of the culture and the accepted focal point is when one defeats another in an argument. Arab culture relishes such practices as accepted norms of society. It is verbal judo, and whoever has the ability to give more verbal punches, wins the battle. The winner then has some fame in the community. The debate is not about debating a thought or an idea; it is a way the individual shows that he can "beat up" the other party and verbally triumph over him.

Mubalkah, which means exaggeration, is another important part of language use for the Arab. For any event that occurs, Arabs are inclined to exaggerate; that can be considered a form of art and verbal skills. However, in the process the truth may be lost. The phenomenon has colored the Arab culture for many areas; it is a part of almost any conversation. Consequently, one has to sift through what is said in order to find the truth or actual occurring events.

Sometimes feelings toward one another can be exaggerated, as well. This dilutes any real feeling between people, resulting in a distorted picture of an entire encounter, due to Mubalkah.

Other influences of the psychology of language in Arab culture include the "magical power of words". Anything they name means it will take place or it will happen. Words are used to curse people or things and Arabs have a strong belief these curses will come true. Sometime they must speak carefully, because one's words may have detrimental effects on others. For example, if a person tells another, "I hope you get sick," then the individual receiving that wish may feel that he will get sick, and it becomes a self-fulfilling wish. The entire Arab culture accepts the omnipotence of words. A word is very powerful and when a person utters words, he feels empowered by the use of the spoken word alone; he does not need to follow his words with actions.

Arab culture is gifted with the manipulation of the language, and it can be considered the backbone of the culture. Sometimes there are some complications with language, as if walking in a labyrinth. The fear of honest expression in the Arab culture can make a person unclear in what he says; therefore, the language can be symbolic in some instances. On the other hand, there sometimes is a hidden meaning to the message and an outsider may find it difficult to understand.

In a distant time, poetry played a major role in the psychology of the tribe; it was and still is one of the few means of self-expression. Each tribe had one poet to protect the tribe, and attack opposing tribes. The poet was held with great regard in the life of the tribe. He was and is the voice defending the honor of the tribe or family. People may fear him because of his sharp tongue and acid language, used to inflict damage on others. Yes, language can cause some damage merely by the speaker fabricating an event or rumor and attaching it to an opponent, thereby putting that opponent on the defensive. Poets can ruin the reputation of other tribes just by spreading rumors, and that keeps opposing tribes busy defending themselves.

Arab people value the Arabic language highly and the lyrics of poetry or songs can soothe their souls. However, if an outside observer listens to Arabic songs, it is very evident that most of lyrics of Arabic songs are sad and depressing. It is a clear representation of the psychology of the culture (mainly Iraqi songs), because Arabs historically have endured much humiliation and suppression. These songs are then historical records of their painful lives.

Arab individuals can be very creative and artistic in the use of language; a certain amount of sharpness characterizes the culture. Language is a primary means of expression, and Arabs use it to the best of their ability. It is also a psychological catharsis for their frustration and disappointment in themselves and others.

Sometimes Arab individuals appear to be vague in expression; it is very difficult to pin them down. Because of persecution, they have written wonderful poetry, but in many instances, only the poet knows the meanings behind his writing. Arab people love symbolic expression; there is no clarity because they do not want others to completely understand them. This experience can be a mystical one and is highly appreciated in the culture.

Arabs are fascinated by flights of fancy and fantasy, because their reality is a bitter one. Thus, one of the best pieces of literature produced by Arabs and given to the world is "One Thousand and One Nights". It is all fantasy. This fascination could be due to the domination of the brain's right hemisphere, which is the one responsible for fantasy/fancy and creativity.

The Arabic language inherited great literature over the centuries. Unfortunately, most of it is complimentary and praises ruthless rulers, because those rulers used to buy poets and writers and pay them handsomely. Thus if translated to other languages, people do not enjoy it, because it is mostly fabrication and lies to ingratiate the author with the rulers. However, if Shakespeare is translated to other languages, everyone around the world enjoys it, because it was written for average people. Thus, sadly, Arabic literature is not suitable for the culture of democracy.

Arabic literature belongs only to the elite class in Arab society, because they have bribed writers to write positive prose and poetry, and make the rulers seem as God's gift to the people. These authors and poets try to represent oppression as something wonderful; in other words, they make the poison of the rulers seem like honey for the masses. What a ridiculous mistake Arab writers have committed, allowing themselves to be tools at the hands of despots!

Arabs vacillate between the love for their language, and the desire to use English in formal correspondence. For them English represents superiority, and is the language of modern science. They view a person who uses a foreign language such as English as somehow a more sophisticated and proud person. There is no clear Arab identity, as in Korea, where all the sciences are taught in their own language.

In several Arab countries, the formal language of correspondence is English, along with French, which is mainly used in North African countries. This can be very disheartening for most Arab intellectuals, who consider the use of Arabic as a stepping-stone for any national development. Ironically, the Arabs are in a serious dilemma in that they are not using Arabic fully, nor are they able to master English. They are in between, and that can lead to stagnation in their national development. Either Arabs must implement Arabic in every sector of the sciences, or master English enough so they can move forward. This issue is beyond the scope of this book, so it is just mentioned here.

Chapter Seventeen

Social Cognitive Learning Theory of the Arab

In their concept of Social-Cognitive Theory, Albert Bandura and other theorists focus on social learning behavior using the modeling process. This method involves an observer and a model; the observer imitates the model. Of course, how well this works depends on a host of factors. For example, people with low self-esteem will more assiduously follow an individual they perceive as having high status. In addition, incompetent people are inclined to model other incompetents; doing so brings some psychological comfort and a false sense of belonging. This imitation of other people's actions, whether incidental or intentional, is the foundation of social learning theory. In effect, learning is at the mercy of societal approval and social reinforcements.

Personal standards are acquired through inference or observational learning, especially from significant figures in one's life, because people do not live in isolation. It is clearly seen how this process of modeling is embedded in Arab society.

Unfortunately, in the Arab world many persons model after leaders or social figures, the head of the office, the head of the tribe or even the head of an organization. Consequently, we may see many "carbon copies" wandering Arab streets. Often, to outside observers the serious inquiry is, why do Arabs have such large numbers of people imitating each other; where is the originality of a person?

Almost the entire society imitates one another without a shred of thought. Of course, this is encouraged quite a bit, and society does not allow people to follow their own path and be unique. Uniqueness is not favored or appreciated in general Arab culture. The opposite is encouraged; if one is dull and follows others like a sheep then he is strongly rewarded by society. Uniqueness is considered a threat to the cohesiveness of society. Arab society encourages conformity and complete submission to established roles and regulations, whether they be written or non-written. The cultural codes should not be violated by members of the culture.

For example, people must wear the same clothes, eat the same food, and use the same conversational language. It's as if when you are among people, you feel each one of them is a copy of all the others, echoing the same messages [As if the whole society is infected with the echomimia or echolalia syndromes]. Individuals will undoubtedly receive compliments for being a "sheep in the herd". The educational system is built on the principle of conformity; do what others do, and do not stray from the main course of society.

In such a case, this kind of modeling can massacre any glimpse of creativity or innovation in the Arab world. Thus, Arab society is lagging behind the progress of the human community.

There is also vicarious modeling. For example, if one sees aggressive behavior or opportunistic attitudes that were rewarded by society, then that vicariously reinforces his modeling. The best example is when people imitate aggressive leaders, or they imitate corrupt governmental officials, because they see the immediate rewards given to those people by society, which fears or avoids them. In the Arab community, on both a small and a large scale, the model has control over the future resources of the observer.

Arab individuals are torn among many systems to emulate. These systems are all operating at the same time: the educational system, the tribal system, the social system and, of course, the family system. To navigate through them all, these systems collectively force the individual to be a blind imitator.

Furthermore, there is an inner struggle for any Arab individual to cope with the colossal demands of external systems, versus internal personal demands, wishes, desires and aspirations. All of these struggles between conflicted forces result in an individual who is non-assertive, weak, angry, frustrated, aggressive, and lacks the ability to reason logically.

Unfortunately, Arab society has worked hard through the years to produce a person who is shallow with a low self-concept. Consequently, people are alike and no one is different than the others. They even use the same vocabularies in daily conversations. Thus, initiating a change in Arab society can be a very remote goal that is hard to achieve, because it may require courage to face an inordinate amount of pressure from society.

The other component of social learning is reinforcement; society reinforces the individual in thinking within the box. Arabs must be submissive in their attitudes and norms of behavior. Thus, there is a shadow person with an absence of real individuality, because the tyranny of the group is the dominant force. If a person has no individuality, undoubtedly there will also be no personal responsibility. This is why people attack public places, because they feel they do not belong to them, and they are not responsible for protecting those amenities.

Living under such a system, people exist only; they are not allowed to discover themselves. People do not drive their concept from within. Thus, the results are violence and aggression toward oneself as well as toward one another.

Of course, the rulers are the primary objects of modeling behavior. Hence, the focal point in this social learning theory: Arabs witness daily the hostile relationship between rulers and the people. That can be one of the underlying causes of most of the dysfunctions/neuroses in Arab society. People learn hostility and internalize it, then project it back on follow members of society. Eventually, the entire society is recycling the painful reality and spreading it among its members.

Chapter Eighteen

The Psychology of Defense Mechanisms In Arab Daily Lives

Arabs are not unique in using some defense mechanisms; most of the people on earth use all kinds of defense mechanisms when faced with and overwhelmed by anxiety. However, there are some defenses used uniquely in some cultures, due to the psychological structure of the whole society. The most common defense mechanisms used in Arab society are:

Frightening Others. The individual may suffer from many fears because of daily threats received from rulers or from the domination of social roles and cultural practices. In response, individuals try to assuage their fears by frightening others; to calm one's anxiety; he must try to frighten others.

Splitting. Arabs look at things from 2 sides only: bad or good; evil or benevolent; black or white; with me or against me. There is no gray area in Arab judgment. As indicated in a previous chapter, Arabs are extreme people in their emotional expression. The color of their judgment is clearly defined. There is no space for maneuvering; there is rigidity in their perception of the world. Perhaps that rigidity comes from the way that individuals have been raised by the family. It is a very primitive defense mechanism, usually used by immature members of society; there is no mental sophistication within those using splitting as a defense mechanism.

Reaction formation. One defense mechanism overused in Arab daily transactions is reaction formation. This involves conspicuously substituting behavior, thoughts or feelings opposite to unacceptable ones. For example, a friend who resents you constantly interferes in your life, in the name of love. Or a religious man shouts about being faithful to God, and asks people to adhere to religious practices, while in his private life he practices the opposite of what he preaches. A person may invite you over for dinner in his house and appear to be close friend, but in reality does not like you, or even cannot stand you. Of course, he does this because he needs you.

Because society has been built on the need for each other, government institutions are not strong enough to ensure the needs of its citizens, or secure equity among people in society. Another possible explanation for reaction formation is because people must hide what they like, or wish to have, or to do in their private lives, to avoid judgment by others. This judgment can be very harsh or extreme, or even may lead to assassination of character without mercy. Thus, psychologically, people have to present the opposite of their inner desires.

Projection. Projection occurs when an individual "puts" the unwanted part of himself on others, because he is unable to tolerate what is inside him/her. Often one may hear in daily conversation how bad other people are; Arabs always put someone down to lift themselves up. A girl, who hates her classmates, may convince herself they hated her first; this is an archaic way of thinking.

However, the more severe form of projection is **Projection Identification**. When others are brutal with him, then he will be brutal with himself; he internalizes the negative messages that come to him, and he behaves accordingly. That is what has happened in the Arab psyche.

Sadistic-masochistic tendencies. Undoubtedly, there is serious flirtation with those tendencies, taking place between the rulers and the people. It's as if the message from rulers is, "Since I am the ruler who knows what is good for you, I have to be brutal with you. That is for your personal benefit; therefore, you have to identify with my brutality. Reactivate your masochist tendencies (the need to be punished) so we can both dance harmoniously." The old wisdom clearly stated that people can be active participants in forming the psychological makeup of their despotic leaders. (For example, the Libyan people have been under Gadaffi's rule for more than four decades, even though he has shown them all kinds of brutality and savagery). There is a saying in the Arab world that the people are the ones who sculpt the psychology of their leaders. Moreover, a tenet of family therapy is that **we teach other how we want to be treated**. The Arab people have participated in the formation of their despotic rulers by being apathetic and obsequious. Overall, it is a dance, and it takes two people to dance, in this case the victim and the victimizer. Undoubtedly, the Arab people bear some of the guilt for their own contributions to their suffering, by allowing despots to rule them for such a long time.

Conformity. Conformity is another part of the neurotic mechanism to escape the insecurity that the Arab has faced for a long time. Since the Arab culture is a collectivist culture, then conformity is something highly valued, because it moves the masses smoothly with less objection to the status quo. However, complaints about the status quo are prevalent in Arab culture, but usually these complaints are only to "vent". This is why the individual Arab is lost in the midst of such confusion.

Identifications with hostile forces. This is self-explanatory—the identification with hostile forces around someone. For example the **Stockholm syndrome** can be seen in the daily lives of the Arab individual. (If the reader is not familiar with this concept, this was when an assault took place on a bank in the capital of Sweden and the employees of the bank were taken as hostages. When the police raided the bank to free the hostages after few weeks, the first ones to fight the police were the employees of the bank.) If an individual is subjugated for a period of psychological or physical abuses, then he may later identify with the abuser or the oppressor. Identifying with hostile forces makes a person borrow certain prestige, or self-esteem, as well as assuaging overwhelming anxiety with which he is faced.

For years, the Arab people have been subjugated to all sorts of abuses and oppressions. Thus, they identify with the hostile forces that surround them, in order to cope with the daily threat in their lives. Demonstrations on Arab city streets supporting the rulers lead outsiders to think that people are in love with their oppressor. The reality is, they demonstrate not out of love but out of sheer fear in order to avoid any harm that may come to them if they do not go to the streets.

Displacement. Since Arabs are abused by each other, they all displace anger at each other. Sometimes they use displacement on a large scale, toward an outside force. Take, for example, when Arabs displace their anger and hostility toward the Western world instead of toward each other. Since they are unable to direct their hostility to their authority figures, they pick a safe object for their hostility; "the West" is safe and anonymous. In addition, antagonistic attitudes prevail in Arab psychology. It is common to see a case of displacement within the family, when the male feels treated unfairly by the outside world. He may bring that attitude home and focus it on the weakest link in the family, which is usually a female member.

Compromise formation. This is a silly defense mechanism. One gives a compliment to another that contradicts attitude or behavior. This can be a result of an inadequate superego development, which leads people to have many types of immature defense mechanisms. For example, you may say to your friend, "You really look so good today", but in reality, you do not like him or he may not look good at all. In effect, you are saying the opposite of your intention.

Denial. Denial is a primitive defense mechanism in which an individual protects himself against threats from the environment by refusing to recognize their existence. Denial is the landmark of Arab psychology; Arabs deny reality and pretend they do not see a particular situation. Of course, there are all kinds of rationalizations or justifications for their denial, which are not necessarily rational or logical. Again, since reality is harsh and bitter, it is better to deny it altogether rather then deal with it and bear pain & suffering.

Humor. One of the most interesting mechanisms used by the Arab is humor. Often, humor can be an expression of hidden anger, or can be used as an outlet for pent up frustration and disappointment. Or in other instances a hostile person is unable to say what is in his mind toward another individual, so he uses humor as a cover up for his hostility. Hence humor may make a hostile tone appear to be less harsh or sound less critical of others. The core of the problem here is lack of assertiveness which leads to such behavior. Overall, Arab society needs to do some hard work to train itself to be more assertive and direct in thinking.

Undoing. Arab culture is well known for using ritualistic behavior, because of superstitions and fictional thoughts. Arab lives are surrounded by shifting sand, not allowing them to be serene and secure. Desert life is filled with superstitious practices. Superstitious persons act from an undesirable impulse, and may make amends by performing some action that nullifies the undesirable action. It may sound irrational but the practice of undoing can rectify a situation psychologically, according to personal belief.

Regression. When the ego is threatened, a person may revert to a more infantile form of behavior as a means to cope with stress. This is regression. There are many examples daily in the lives of Arabs, such as an adult throwing a temper tantrum, or breaking things around the house. These behaviors are seen as a regression.

Ambivalence. Often, the Arab may suffer from a great deal of ambivalence about many things in his life. It is mixed feelings toward others and often can alternate between love and hate; anger and peace; or agreement and disagreement. Ambivalence causes frustration, as a person is not being able to think or feel clearly. This psychological state can be attributed to how the individual was raised, which is to please others at the expense of himself/herself.

Oral fixation. There are two kinds of fixations. The first is caused by growing up with an under-indulgent mother; a mother who has not invested herself in her child. Usually in such cases, adults have aggressive characteristics like envy, manipulation and suspicion of others. The second type of oral fixation is caused from growing up with an overly indulgent mother, who has pampered her child. Usually in this situation adults have characteristics such as gullibility, admiration of others and excessive dependency on others. We find all of these characteristics in the Arab personality. For example, being envious of another is quite common in Arab culture. However, the characteristics caused by an over-indulgent mother are more common in the Arab personality. In general, this personality is gullible and naïve; they believe what authority figures tell them. They also show great admiration of the rulers or the head of any organization. Undoubtedly, that puts them at a disadvantage, giving the rulers multiple opportunities to take advantage of them.

Sublimation. Sublimation is a form of displacement in which a socially acceptable goal replaces one that is unacceptable. For example, it is very common for people to attempt to overcome their primitive impulses by being deeply involved in religion. An athlete may be someone who is trying to triumph over his aggressive tendencies by participating in sports.

Persona. Carl Jung came up with this concept, which is compromise between the demands of the environment and the necessities of the individual inner constitution. It is the mask worn to function adequately in the world. People hide their real selves behind masks. People may exhibit this mask while they are in the mosque/church, among a group, where they work, or even with their family. Often there is even a mask for every place and every occasion.

The shadow. Again, Jung indicated this is the personification of evil within the psyche of every one of us; i.e., the devil in various forms. Some may never bring themselves to confront absolute evil within their depths. This shadow exists in all of us and manifests itself in two forms in Arab culture. 1) Arabs have urges toward self-destruction, which can be an unconscious tendency. 2) There is a desire to harm others. This desire can be the more pronounced of the two, and is often seen in the daily lives of the Arab society.

Undoubtedly, when a person grows up in an unhealthy and threatening environment, where parents are harsh and critical, or society demands complete submission to its neurotic tyrannical practices, the growth of that individual is likely to be stifled or stunted. That may lead an individual to repress evil forces within the psyche. One day these forces will erupt without warning, to uncover a personality that has many psychological cracks. Moreover, individuals under these circumstances feel helpless and castrated. Such individuals may become also outraged, and will direct their frustration and anger toward society at large, because they feel that their community, society or family have contributed to make them a psychologically impotent human being.

In conclusion, there are several reasons why people use defense mechanisms. 1) These mechanisms manifest to assuage overwhelming anxiety that Arabs tend to face in their daily lives. 2) Defense mechanisms alleviate Arabs' suffering and 3) protect their fragile Egos. Defense mechanisms can also 4) hide some evil part of the personality or 5) assist the Arab to manage/ negotiate his world as best he can. Moreover, the Arab people in particular may suffer from an infantile personality, because they are fixated on the oral stages of development as defined by Freud. This is why Arabs have love affairs with food, and explains the fascination with language idioms. Most of all this explains the submission to the father figure in their lives, which in the Arab's case, is the ruler.

Chapter Nineteen

The Psychology of Stigmatizations In Arab Culture

There are a few stigmas in the Arab culture; the first stigma is **illness**. This does not refer to every illness, but primarily refers to epilepsy. If a woman has epileptic seizures, her chance of marriage can suffer. This is why she hides her illness. It is the same with men, but with less severity. It is considered the work of *jinn* or an evil spirit who possesses the body of the person, thus, the "fit" or attack. Undoubtedly, modern medicine has treatment for these seizures and they can be controlled by medication and/ or surgery. However, the fear of disclosing this kind of illness inevitably reduces the marriageability of the woman. Although some people may take that chance and marry a woman with seizures, it is rare.

What is the analytical view for such stigma? Arab culture has some elements of superstition, perhaps due to the uncertainty of desert life. When the society shifted to an agricultural basis, the stigma toward illness became more pronounced, because a man always looks to marry a strong woman, who can give him healthy boys to work on the farm or in the fields. Interestingly,

Arab society prefers plump, chubby women over thin ones, because they think plump women may produce healthy babies.

Mental illness can also carry a serious stigma. Thus, the family tends to hide it, or the person may claim that he has a physical illness instead. Consequently, psychosomatic symptoms are more prevalent in Arab culture than in others. A sick person can more easily say, "I have stomach pain", rather than "I am depressed". Society may accept stomach pain as normal but depression can be the work of evil and is not accepted by the average Arab. This is why in almost any clinic in the Arab world there are serious cases of somatizations.

Nevertheless, in cases of serious mental illness like schizophrenia or paranoia, the family may keep the afflicted family member at home, and is unwilling to let others know about him/her. They fear that the stigma maybe become attached to the whole family. They also see this kind of illness as a punishment from God or a possession of evil spirits. Thus, they have to keep the ill person away from the eyes of others.

A second stigma prevailing in Arab culture for many years is **the Sharif**, or female sexuality. The reputation of the family honor is at stake. If a woman has sex or loses her virginity, that can bring unbearable damage to the entire family. Society considers it a black stain on the family's image. That probably will also affect her sister's matrimonial future, as it is a matter of losing face and a place in society. For a woman in Arab culture, staying a virgin until after marriage is the ultimate honor for the family. To the outside observer, it seems that Arab culture is obsessed with female sexuality. Put into historical perspective, however, it can clearly be understood. Arabs are nomadic tribes, who previously would raid each other and take women as hostages along with the livestock. The women were abused sexually, so the Arab developed sensitivity toward that, always wanting to keep women away from intruders or predators.

Working in certain **professions** can carry a stigma. For example, those who shine or repair shoes are viewed by society with some disdain. A plumber, who works in fixing bathrooms, may be stigmatized, and will have a hard time finding a wife. If he has children, they will suffer. Another stigmatized profession is that of a porter. People in this profession normally do not marry from society unless it is from within their own group of people. Society looks down at the *Mehinah*, the Arabic word literally meaning demeaning job or profession. **Poverty** can be a stigma as well. Arab society looks at the poor with less respect than the rich, and poverty is considered a social stigma. Society sees them as unfortunate people, and psychologically speaking, people do not like to be around unfortunate persons. Conversely, many people like to be around the rich, because they think it might "rub off" on them. Arabs think if you associate with successful people then you are successful, and if you associate with failures then you are a failure, too.

The psychological explanation for these professions being the target of disrespect is because the tribal system does not appreciate hard labor. This is a holdover from the desert concept. Yet, it is a most fascinating phenomenon that the Arab world suffers from a very high rate of unemployment, while the Arab world is one of the highest employers of workers "imported" from outside the Arab world.

In general, Arabs do not like to do hard jobs, and they are too proud to perform any job they consider a low-grade profession. Perhaps they are lazy, yet if they immigrate to another country, they will work any job. For example, the Lebanese do not like to work as gas station attendants in Lebanon, but they will work in that job and all kinds of other jobs when they go to another country. It does not make sense, but that is the reality.

Another primary stigma is **physical handicaps**. Sadly, Arab families also like to keep the physically handicapped at home and do not take them out to public places. Again, they feel it is revenge from God for a misdeed that family member may have committed. This is a punishment for them. Unfortunately, the handicapped are seldom viewed by the community.

As far as psychological explanations to these other stigmas, the Arab culture is an old culture. Normally old cultures tend to inherent accumulations of outdated values, roles and practices.

The Indian culture shares many stigmas with the Arab culture, because it is an old culture as well, with stifling practices. Some cultures may evolve faster than others. Hopefully Arab culture is moving toward liberating itself from meaningless social practices, and freeing itself from the stigmatizations of illness, honor and hard work.

Chapter Twenty

The Recent Phenomenon of Terrorism in Arab Lives

The Psychology of Extremism

Aggression is a part of the human psychological makeup. We are born with the tendency to be aggressive. Unless we work sincerely to cultivate this tendency, however, how many people are seriously pruning their aggression, and let alone how many people are conscious of their aggression? We occasionally observe a spike of aggression in our daily lives because of some stimulation in our surroundings.

Unfortunately, lately many Arabs blow themselves to pieces in acts of terrorism. This is a new phenomenon to the Arab culture, because the Islamic religion has placed a great premium on human life, and forbids any Muslim to kill himself. So, why do these people resort to such heinous a crime and kill many people along with themselves?

It is a very puzzling phenomenon, and the psychological explanations may be insufficient to adequately analyze it. However, we have to try to understand what is in the mind of the terrorists who disrespect the sanctity of lives in general. It is worth trying to explain this complicated phenomenon from analytical perspectives. Numerous contributing factors may lead an individual to act destructively in this way:

1) These people have developed a mindset of righteousness; they are right in their beliefs, and everybody else is wrong. Since all others are wrong, it is worthwhile to take their lives and make them non-existent.

2) They have developed a sense of guardianship. They feel they are responsible for society and, since society is going in a different direction from their own direction, they feel they have the complete right to correct that direction by any means, even if they resort to taking lives.

3) Their minds are diluted by poisonous ideas. They feel the world is a bad and terrible place to live, thus their personal message is that they have to end their lives and the lives of others, and look forward to life in Heaven.

4) Often, they come from a very disturbed background. They may have seen a lot of abuse in their family or in their community, which helped foster their negative outlook toward themselves and toward society.

5) They are very illogical or irrational beings to start with, and have very twisted views of the world around them. Thus, they can justify their killing of others.

6) They may have a very harsh superego that tends to always cause them pain. By doing something radical, either killing themselves or others, they lessen the pressure of the superego.

7) Possibly, they suffer from the meaninglessness in their lives, and overwhelming existential anxiety is taking over their conscious and subconscious mind.

8) These people have serious pathological anger for which they are unable to find an outlet other than through revenge toward society. Society at large becomes the object of their hostility.

9) They have been indoctrinated with many false beliefs, and are cognitively vulnerable and impressionable. It is

very hard for them to give up these beliefs, so they act upon them.

10) These terrorists are gullible and naïve; they do not have sophisticated views, and do not question the authority figures who indoctrinated them. Often, they do not have the capacity to question or examine what has been given to them. In other words, they accept everything wholesale.

11) These people could also suffer from a cognitive deficit, and mentally the appreciation for life does not exist in their personal lives.

12) Doubtless, they do not have a nurturing mother in their lives; they grow up very dry and cold emotionally. Thus, death does not mean anything to them, because they consider themselves already dead.

13) They may suffer a lot set backs and failure in their lives, and thus have developed tremendous hate for themselves and society. Therefore, death for them can be a means to an end . . . the end of the psychological pain they have inside.

14) This fatalistic tendency can be also a case of the Sadomasochist dynamic: I inflect pain on people and in return, they inflict pain on me. It can be the ultimate sadomasochist fulfillment.

15) Such people lack a real faith in God; there is a hole in their soul. They are in constant pain because of that spiritual void. Undoubtedly, if they had love for God in their hearts, or they had love for themselves, they would not take their lives in their hands. They could also have a very shallow or superficial understanding of Islam. Faith in the Almighty God is guaranteed to invigorate the spirit of the individual. This faith makes them overflow with love for every living or non-living thing in the universe. Sadly, they may see religion from their own shallow perspective, as just an empty ritualistic behavior.

16) There is a serious case of mental limitation as far as these people are concerned. Either they do not have, or they do not use their mental capabilities like the rest of us to improve the quality of their lives.

17) There is an absence of a loving relationship in their lives, because love can brighten up their lives and bring joy to their existence.

18) They may have been using drugs for a while, and thus cannot rationalize or have a balanced view of the world around them.

19) Hard people to deal with, they are stubborn and defiant in their nature. Thus, this rigidity in their personality may cause them to carry out such crimes.

20) They may have a serious case of poor self-image. They do not value themselves highly; on the contrary, they view themselves as a useless soul. Death for them can be a solution to their nagging self-loathing.

21) Finally, the **Thanatos** tendency (the desire to destroy and perish) is highly active within their psyche, according to Freud. This is as opposed to the **Eros** tendency, which is the desire to live and build. It seems there is no trace of Eros in their psyche.

We also see some hostility toward the West. That is possibly the result of the frustration of the Arab masses, which has developed through the years. Western rulers always stand beside and support some of the Arab despotic rulers, even though the Arab sees the West preaching democracy. This stance by Western governments can make the Arabs angry and frustrated, through the years this anger has turned to hostility toward the West.

Unfortunately, the West does not understand this rather obvious fact; often the West fuels this hostility more by further supporting the despotic rulers in the Arab world. The Foreign Minster of France, Alain Juppe, in his last interview with BBC acknowledged that the West always looks for the stability of Arab regimes, and has ignored the plight of the Arab people and their desire for freedom.

In conclusion, if someone has a conversation with these people (terrorists), you hear many illogical and poisonous thoughts, which have contributed to their cognitive rigidity and black and white thinking. Their attitudes are, "If you are not with my logic then you are against me, and I am entitled to take your lives away, and eliminate your existence".

This very dangerous phenomenon has appeared on the world stage lately. It needs to be addressed collectively by human society, because the mission of these people is to create death and destruction. Our modern civilization is faced with a serious challenge, in that extremism has one goal: to kill and destroy what mankind has built over hundreds of years.

Then what is the answer to such an imminent challenge? It's unfortunately not that simple, but we may need to go to the roots of the problem to eradicate it, and we should not entertain any short-term solutions because short-term solutions tend to be short-lived.

Although I have personally offered some analytical views of the causes of terrorism, the effective solution to such a mammoth problem is beyond the scope of this book.

Chapter Twenty One

The Recent Developments In the Arab World

Clearly, 2011 is the year of Arab revolutions, and the year of sudden transformations in the psyche of the Arab people. It is fascinating that there has been continuing revolution in Arab countries. First Tunisia, then Egypt, Yemen, Libya, and now Syria, all on a large scale, while there have been small-scale revolutions in other Arab States. There are several analytical-psychological explanations:

1) Let us refer to the Koshima research regarding monkeys on a few islands in Japan. The phenomenon was quite puzzling and enigmatic. There are monkeys who live on a few scattered islands in Japan, and the Japanese government feeds them by dropping potatoes to them from helicopters. The potatoes reach the ground and mix with sands; normally the monkeys eat the potatoes without washing the sand from them in the nearby sea.

    One day a young monkey took a potato and washed it in the seawater. Suddenly, the whole tribe of monkeys started to wash their potatoes in the seawater before eating them. The first monkey who initiated washing the potatoes transferred the particular task or change in the mental level to the other monkeys on other islands. Even though they have not witnessed the potato washing, it was transferred through the collective consciousness to all of the monkeys, on an unconscious level. Currently, when potatoes are thrown to them, they go right away to the sea and wash them. They have learned from each other through the collective consciousness. This case was well-researched and documented. This is perhaps what has happened in the Arab psyche; there was a collective consciousness about breaking the chain of fear, and revolt against the despotic rulers began. Is it possible the change that started in Tunisia has transferred to the rest of Arab world?

2) There has been a paradigm shift in the behavior of people. Old patterns of behavior have been broken, and people no longer see life as worth living. Actually, they have felt dead anyway, so why not try to die with some dignity? Death is less frightening now than it used to be. Consequently, they went to the streets in huge masses, facing imminent death, but they did not care. The entire world has been stunned by the bravery of the masses, and the audacity of the people, especially the ruthless leaders.

3) Another possible reason for these recent developments is that the Arab people have reached "critical mass", like in physics, in their collective consciousness. They will no longer tolerate their long-standing abuse by the rulers; it created a morphogenetic field making the change accessible.

4) There was a domino effect, similar to what happened in Eastern Europe in the mid-1990s. One block fell and the rest followed, which gave people the impetus for change. Nothing can stop such change. Despots around the world have the same concept for ruling people: treat people like bacteria. Use antibiotics as much as you can to kill the bacteria. Use force and be as brutal as possible to kill the souls of the people. However, people in such a situation

become more defiant, and force can no longer silence them.

5) Another aspect here is the psychology of downtrodden people who have reached the peak of helplessness and hopelessness. Suddenly, they pick themselves up and dust themselves off from the years of abuse, and turn into a roaring lion. Human history has shown us myriad examples of such cases. The Arab people have been kicked and beaten up psychologically for a long time, and it seems the voice of revenge is coming from inside them to face what has happened to them.

6) What has happened recently in the Arab world is a massive internal shift in the psyche of people. Fear no longer controls them, because there is nothing left to fear: no jobs for the youth, poor infrastructure, poor educational systems, poor health systems, lack of justice, constant abuse by rulers, and, most of all, lack of respect for the wishes of and expression by the populace.

7) The recent developments in the Arab world are similar to the myth of the Phoenix, which exists in folklore in almost every culture around the world. The Phoenix was burned by fire and reduced to ashes, but came back to live and gave rebirth to himself. The Arab people have been burned savagely by the fire of their pathological rulers. Now they are coming back, giving rebirth to themselves like the young phoenix born anew from its ashes and come to live again. Undoubtedly, the soul of the Arab people has been resurrected, enabling them to break the chain of fear that has shackled them for many centuries.

Overall, we are witnessing history in the making. Most disheartening are the reactions of the despotic rulers to the change. Sadly, they have shown their ultimate brutality and hatred of their own people. The rulers' message, in every country where revolution has taken root, is very clear: "either I rule over you or I have to eliminate you or wipe you off the face of the earth". Literally, they have destroyed their countries, and they are willing to kill anyone who opposes them or take revenge on those who revolt against them. It is very shameful to see that, and the entire world watches the atrocity unfold every day in a different part of the Arab world.

The behavior of the Arab rulers in facing recent uprisings or revolutions has shown no shortage of pathological leaders such as Saddam, Gadaffi, Ben Ali, Saleh of Yemen, Bashar of Syria and Mubarek of Egypt. They are the embodiment of Evil. They have shown they actually hate their people with a passion, and they are thirsty to shed blood . . . anyone's. Undoubtedly, they have antisocial personality disorders, as one of the characteristics of antisocial personality disorder is killing without remorse. Humanity has seen these faces before, as with Hitler in 20th century Germany. They will not hesitate to kill the last person in the country just to rule.

There is a fascinating proverb in Arabic: **Alemarah walo ala Alhejarah**. The literal translation is: "ruling over even a heap of stones is better then not ruling". It is clear; Arabs like to govern over people. Perhaps that is part of human psychology, as with the desire for power and prestige. However, in the Arab culture this has been more drastic because the average individual has a low self-concept, including rulers. Ruling others can give some psychological fulfillment to their dwarfed Egos.

Conclusions

There are a few observations that can be summarized after reading this book. It can be of value for future applications as well as for improvement of existing conditions.

People in general are like plants; they take from the earth the nutrients suitable to their structures. Thus, Arab behavior is a product of the circumstances that surround them, and if we need different behaviors then we have to change the circumstances.

1) Cutting dead branches from a tree does not make the tree healthy; perhaps we need to change the soil. A total transformation to the entire existing archaic system in the Arab world may be needed on many levels. For instance, the educational system, family scripts and, most of all, the governmental systems need to be overhauled. The government has to be democratic rather than run by a bunch of despots who rule forever.

2) The majority of Arabs are fascinated, consciously or unconsciously, with the **cult of personality**. Everyone wants to have an idol to worship or glorify. Such disorder has been practiced for many, many years, and it seems to be indelible in the Arab's neurons. Arabs are also inclined to assign a certain amount of holiness to their "chosen people" and they become enamored of them. Undoubtedly, those chosen people, whether they are governmental rulers, religious figures, head of an organization or the head of a community, will abuse their power and position and eventually will cause a lot of pain and suffering.

It is disheartening to see that; perhaps the soil of the Arab world is fertile for growing dictators. It may have the necessary nutrients for the growth of dictators, because the Arab people throughout history have produced in abundance the most brutal, callous dictators in the history of mankind. Fortunately, today we are witnessing the demise of those dictators. However, the damage is done; they have held the Arab back. They let Arab society fall behind the progress of the human community, even though they have huge reservoirs of natural resources, and sit on some of the most valuable real estate on earth. The only salvation from such destructive trends is the total emancipation of the Arab soul from the cult of personality, or idol worship.

3) Women in the Arab world must be treated with respect and appreciation, rather than as a threat to male members of society. The female has to have a good foundation of self-esteem in order to rear a generation of healthy children, rather then cripple them psychologically.

4) Arabs also have been obsessed with female sexuality. We can understand that from a historical perspective, when tribes raided each other in the desert. They took women as well as livestock and abused the women. It seems however that even in modern times Arabs are unable to transcend the historical practice and look at female sexuality as something private and more of a biological matter. They still attach a certain degree of holiness to female sexuality. Unfortunately, men always assume devious intentions and mistrust when it comes to women, and that puts women in a defensive posture most of the time. In such situations, society loses tremendous energy, which could normally be channeled for the good of society.

5) There is a serious conflict in the Arab psyche between Bedouins values and Islamic values. The Bedouin values encourage pride, selfishness, greed, violation of others, and the use of force to settle conflicts. Islamic values focus on helping each other, being human, settling conflicts by the law of God, taking care of the needy and the weak in

society, respecting the sanctity of life and being humble. The conflict exists in all levels of society, and the main reason for such conflict is that the Arab has not absorbed the true teaching of God, but instead focuses on the **ritualistic practices of religion**. Sadly, the **Jahelia values are in force** [time before Islam]. At present what the Arab needs is to hold onto faith in God, which can enlighten his/her empty heart and free his/her soul from the darkness.

6) The old culture tends to have a lot of do's and don'ts. All of this discipline can be like a steamroller, killing all creativity and generating fears. The Arabs must realize that and free themselves.

7) Since early history, Arabs and Jews were traders; this may explain why the Arab tends to "wheel and deal". They also calculate benefits and losses in their daily transactions. That can have a psychological impact on people's behavior and the way they view the world. Friendship can be the best example. Someone is a friend as long as he benefits from the friendship. Once that benefit is absent, he walks away and casts aside his former "friend". Arab popular songs testify as to the difficulty in finding true and lasting friendships. People often form a relationship based on ulterior motive, not just for the sake of friendship only. Perhaps that is part of human nature.

8) Unfortunately, the Arab world has refused to face up to the challenge that has been presented to it recently, and they use projection as a defense mechanism. They tend to blame everyone else for their own societal ills and never look to themselves and their contributions to their painful reality. Arab rulers blame foreign intervention if any one of their people raises an objection; they never blame their own mismanagement of the country. That has to be understood and changed otherwise Arabs will stay in the same vicious cycle.

9) Assertiveness in Arab culture has not been nurtured; on the contrary, compliance is encouraged. That can have serious psychological ramifications on the individual. It also can breed some neurotic tendencies, as the conflict

builds between societal demands and individual needs and aspirations.

10) The **Wasta** practice, the Arabic word for **favoritism and nepotism**, can be an incurable disease that infects the body of Arab society. It needs to be eradicated; everyone should be treated based on his merits rather than on whom he knows. That is disgraceful to the whole society and people feel bitter about it. Sadly, the entire governmental structure is built on nepotism.

11) The hidden reality is that the world, as we see it around us, is what our past thoughts and experiences have created. If we need or desire a different world, we have to change our thinking to create a fresh, healthy world around us. The Arab culture has inherited a lot of useless practices and meaningless values that do not nurture the creativity of the population.

12) The Arab culture is oppressive, and normally an oppressive culture tends to breed a lot of neuroses, such as mistrust, anger, frustration, and suspicion, not only within the psyche of the individual, but even among family members. People by nature want to be free. Individual freedom is not a luxury; it is a necessity and indispensable for the psychological well-being of every individual in any society.

13) My last conclusion is a recommendation to the human community, [particularly the Arab people]. We have to establish "**human radar**" to watch for any growth of dictators in any part of the world, but mainly the Arab world. If a dictatorship appears, we have to do whatever it may take to prevent such growth. Leaving a dictator to establish himself in any part of the world can have a mammoth cost to the entire human community. It is more dangerous than the tsunami, both in the cost of human lives as well as in the destruction of human civilization.

For example, the dictators of Africa have embezzled all national wealth and left the continent reeling under poverty, wars and diseases. Or in the latest development in Libya, Gaddafi ruled Libya for more than four decades, yet he has not even built a decent hospital in the country. He has squandered the wealth of the people, and when the people revolted again him and wanted to remove him, he engaged them in very destructive war.

In order to avoid such an apocalyptic future from those dictators who are possessed by the demonic power, the human community needs to be watchful. The consequence of dictatorship is immeasurable destructions; it is worse than any epidemic of disease in the world. Moreover, it will have serious ripple effect on every corner on the globe. It is not confined to a specific country, but it will harm the rest of the human community as we saw in the rise of Hitler.

What has brought me to this recommendation is that I am a psychologist who is deeply concerned with the well being of people in any part of the world. I have witnessed the dictators' rules in the Arab world and seen how much damage they have caused. The sad diagnosis for those living under the rule of dictators is depression, anxiety, paranoia, adjustment disorder, psychosomatic illness, and delusional thinking. In summary, the consequences of living under dictators are people who feel worthless, and are deeply troubled psychologically. Thus, they can not offer anything either to themselves or to the human community other than pain and suffering.

References

American Psychiatric Association, (2000).Diagnostic and statistical manual of mental disorders. (4th ed.) Washington, D.C.

Alwardi, A. (1969). Social glimpses of modern Iraq, Palgrave Macmillan.

Alkasmi, A. (2004). Concepts in Arab mind. Casablanca, Morocco. In Arabic.

Abu-Baker, K.(2005).The impact of social values on the psychology of gender among Arab couple. Isr J. Psychiatry Relat. Sci. 42, 106-115.

Ajami, F. (1992).The Arab predicaments. Cambridge University Press.

Bandura, A. (1977). Social learning theory. Englewood Cliffs. N.J. Prentice Hall.

Becker, E.(1971). The birth and the death of meaning. The Free Press, New York.

Bowlby. J. (1982). Attachment and loss. New York, Basic Books.

Burnham, T. & Phelan, J.(2000). Mean genes. Peruses Publication, Cambridge, MA.

Buss, D. (1995). Psychology sex difference origins through sexual selection. American Psychologist. 50 [30]. 164-171.

Butcher. J.N. (1990). MMPI-2 In psychological treatment. New York. Oxford University Press.

Doidge, N.(2007). The brain that change itself. Penguin Book.

Ellis. A. (1974). Rational—emotive theory. Oxford England, Brunner/Mosel.

Ellis, A. & Abrams, M. (2009). Personality theories. Sage publication.Inc.

Erikson. H. (1964). Insight and responsibility, New York. W.W. Norton.

Epstein.(1995). Thoughts without a thinker, Basic books.

Eysenck. H. J. (1967). The biological basis of personality. Springfield, IL.

Fenichel, O. (1945). The psychoanalytic theory of neurosis. W.W. Norton. New York.

Franklin, V. (1997). Man's search for meaning. Basic Books.

Freud. A. (1936). The ego and mechanisms of defense. Madison, CT. International University Press.

Freud, S. (1916). Psychopathology of everyday life. New York: Macumillan.

Freud, S. (1930). A general introduction to psychoanalysis. New York: Horace Liveright.

Freud, S. (1949). On narcissisms: an introduction. New York: Modern Library.

Freud, S. (1949). Three essays on the theory of sexuality. London: Imago.

Freud, S. (1959). Collected papers. New York. Basic Books.

Fromm.E. (1981). To have or to be. Bantam Books, New York.

Fromm, E (1980). The heart of man. HarperCollins.

Fromm, E. (1994). Escape from freedom. Owl Book.

Fromm, E. (2006) Art of loving. Harper Perennial Modern Classics.

Gibran, K. (1923). The prophet. Penguin Books.

Gilbert, D. (2006). Stumbling on happiness. Vintage Books, New York.

Goldman. (2006) Emotional intelligence. New York. Bantam Books.

Greenberg, J. R. & Mitchell, S.A. (1983). Object relation in psychoanalytic theory,
Cambridge, MA; Harvard University press.

Grigg, R. (1989). The Tao of being, Humanics, New age. Atlanta, Georgia.

Heider, J. (1985). The Tao of leadership. Humanics, New age, Atlanta, Georgia.

Hitti, P. K. (1937). History of Arab.

Horney, K. (1937). The neurotic personality of our time. New York; W.W. Norton.

Ibn Khaldoun, (1406). Muqaddimah—Prolegomenon.

James, W. (1905). The principles of psychology. New York: Henry Holt.

Jung, C. (1933). Modern man in search of a soul. London, Kegan Paul.

Jung, C. (1969). The archetype and the collective unconscious. Princeton. NJ: Princeton University Press.

Kafaji, T. (2010). Inward Journey. Authorhouse publishing company, Indiana

Klein, S. (2002). The science of happiness. Marlow & company. New York.

Klein, M. & Riviera, J. (1964). Love, hate, and reparation. New Your: W.W. Norton.

Kohut, H. (1977). The restoration of the self. New York. International Universities Press.

Lazarus, A. (1976). Multimodal behavior therapy. New York. Springer.

Lipton, B.H. (2008). The biology of belief. Hay House, Inc. Carlsbad, California.

Mahler, M. (1971). A study of the separation-individuation process and its possible application to borderline phenomena in the psychoanalytic situation. The psychoanalytic of the child, 26. 403-424.

Maslow. A. (1954). Motivation and personality. New York. Harper.

May, R. (1953). Man's search for himself. New York: W.W. Norton.

May, R. (1969). Love and will. New York.W.W. Norton.

Milgram, S. (1963). Behavior study of obedience. Journal of Abnormal psychology. 63. 371-378.

Milgram, S. (1974). Obedience to authority: An experimental view. New York; Harper & Row.

Mitchell, S. (1988). Tao Te Ching. HarperCollins.

Patai, R. (1970). The Arab mind, Hatherleigh Press.

Pavlov, I. P. (1927). Conditioned reflexes: An investigation of the physiological activity of the cerebral cortex. London: Oxford University Press.

Ricard, M. 2003. Happiness. Little Brown and Company, New York.

Rogers. (1961). On becoming a person: A therapist's view of psychotherapy. Boston: Houghton Mifflin.

Rotter, J. (1954). Social learning and clinical psychology. Englewood Cliffs: Prentice Hall.

Rychman, R. M.(2008). Theories of personality. Thomson & Wadsworth, USA.

Seligman, M. (1975). Generality of learning helplessness in man. Journal of Personality and Social Psychology. 31 2, 311-327.

Seligman, M. (2002). Authentic happiness. New York: Free Press.

Skinner, B.F. (1953). Science and human behavior. New York, Macmillan.

Skinner, B.F. (1971).Beyond freedom and dignity. New York: Knopf.

Watson, J.B. & Rayner, R. (1920). Conditioned emotional reaction. Journal of experimental psychology, 3, 1-14.

Wundt. (1904). Principle of physiological psychology. New York: Macmillan.

www.ingramcontent.com/pod-product-compliance
Lightning Source LLC
Chambersburg PA
CBHW020241290526
45784CB00003B/1060